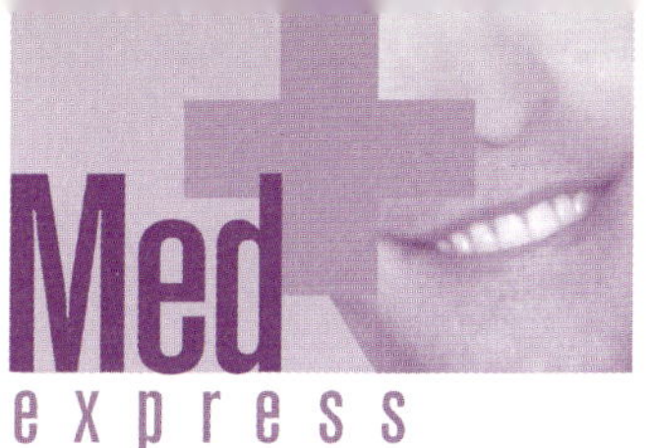


# overcoming fatigue

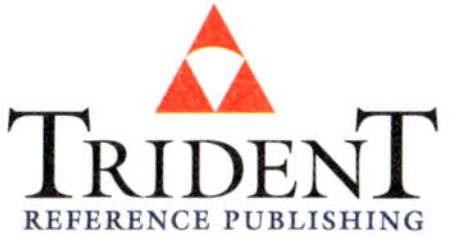

**NOTE**
This publication is intended to provide reference information for the reader on the covered subject. It is not intended to replace personalized medical diagnosis, counseling, and treatment from a doctor or other healthcare professional.
**Before taking any form of treatment you should always consult your physician or medical practitioner.**
The publisher and authors disclaim any liability, loss, injury or damage incurred as a consequence, directly or indirectly, of the use and application of the contents of this book.

Published by:
Tridcnt Reterence Publishing
801 12th Avenue South, Suite 400
Naples, Fl 34102 USA
Phone: + 1 239 649 7077
Email: sales@trident-international.com
Website: www.trident-international.com

Overcoming Fatigue


**Publisher**
Simon St. John Bailey

**Editor-in-chief**
Isabel Toyos

**Art Director**
Aline Talavera

**Photos**
© Trident Reference Publishing, © Getty Images, © Jupiter Images, © Planstock, © J. Alonso

Includes index
ISBN 1582799709 (hc)
UPC 615269997093 (hc)
ISBN 158279958X (pbk)
UPC 615269799581 (pbk)



2005 Edition
Printed in USA

# overcoming fatigue

# Are you excessively tired?

Getting tired is a natural symptom, which is a result of the process of using energy during the day for a number of daily activities. When you are excessively tired, it's good to take a look at your daily tasks and habits. There are also a number of natural remedies that can help to relieve fatigue.

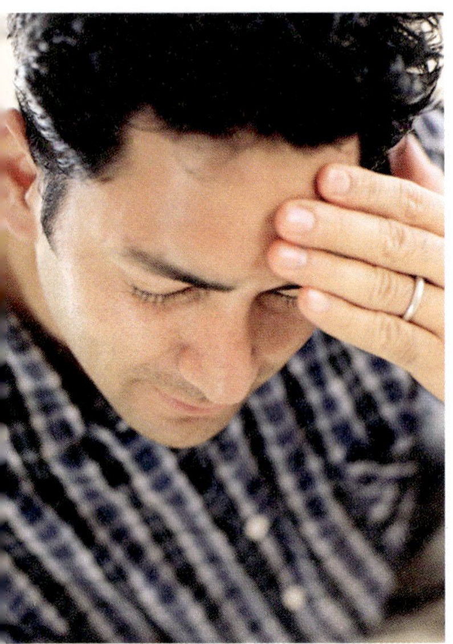

Feeling tired at the end of the day is natural, and can even be a good feeling because it is an indicator that you need to rest and helps you to go to sleep. However, excessive tiredness tends to appear when you have trouble maintaining healthy habits: not getting regular sleep, not exercising regularly, eating an abnormal or unbalanced diet, smoking, not drinking enough liquids or not dedicating enough time to relax and have fun may cause excessive tiredness.

In order for you to recuperate your normal energy level it is fundamental to know how you could change your daily routine to readapt your lifestyle and incorporate healthy habits. In general, it's good to introduce physical exercise into your daily activities, make sure you stick to a sleep routine, eat a balanced diet, with plenty of nutritious foods that are a good source of energy, and stay away from nervous system depressants, such as alcohol and tobacco. Think about what you could change to achieve a more balanced, stress-free lifestyle.

There are also a number of multi-vitamin

supplements and treatments that are very effective in fighting against tiredness when it is triggered by natural causes or lifestyle habits. In this case it is advisable that you take a higher amount of B complex vitamins ($B_1$, $B_6$, $B_{12}$). Vitamins with antioxidant properties, such as vitamins E and C, can also be effective. Multivitamin supplements contain essential amino-acids (magnesium combined with zinc) and other trace minerals such as magnesium and selenium that help your body recuperate when you are excessively fatigued.

## OTHER TIPS IF YOU FEEL TIRED

It is important that you pay attention to symptoms of prolonged tiredness. This means that even though you have a healthy lifestyle, tiredness persists or increases during a week's time. If you find that you feel fatigued for more than 15 days, it's important that you consult your doctor, because it can be a symptom of an illness. If there is no physical cause for prolonged-fatigue, then it may be advisable to see a psychologist because it might be caused by depression. There is another type of fatigue that is worrisome: this occurs in the evening, after a day of normal, light activities and doesn't disappear after a regular night's sleep. When this occurs, medical attention is recommended.

### TO PREVENT GETTING TIRED

To make sure that at the end of the day you aren't excessively tired we've compiled a list of tips so that you can enjoy your leisure time with loved ones:

- Take brief breaks every two hours, especially if your are studying, doing any intellectual task, or working in front of the computer. Stretch out your legs, take a walk and whenever possible, rest your eyes and mind, focusing your attention on the landscape or the view from your room.
- If you work in a closed-in workplace, try to make sure that the space is ventilated so you don't lack oxygen.
- Work in silence or with soft music in the background. Often times, when flooding your sensory perception with information, it is best to avoid the noise of the television and radio or over-stimulating information, while you are working. It is also advised to limit the use of cellular phones.
- Plan out the daily tasks that you need to complete, setting realistic deadlines for the day. This can help you to avoid the tensions that completely exhaust you by the end of the day.
- Eat lunch far away from your workplace and don't take your work with you to lunch . Avoid phone calls and conversations about work during lunch.
- Don't work more than eight hours a day. Reserve private time for yourself and to share with your family and loved ones. This will provide the comfort that you need to fully rest, recharge positive energy and start the next day energized and with enthusiasm.

# How to fight fatigue

If simple lifestyle changes and not physical illnesses cause fatigue, there are a number of alternative therapies that can help you to beat tiredness.

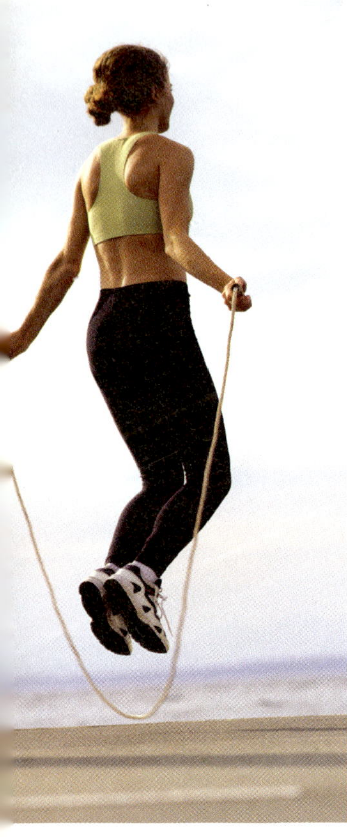

You can begin to overcome your tiredness with some simple measures:

- **Eat well.** Your diet should be balanced and include the principle foods in the food pyramid: lean meats, fruit, vegetables, cereals and low-fat dairy. In addition, it is good to drink 6 to 8 glasses of water a day. Drinking water and fruit juice are important because a lack of liquids and minerals can make you fatigued.
- **Improve your physical activity.** An exercise routine can be very helpful to help you recuperate your energy. It is recommended to start an exercise program with the supervision of your doctor.
- **Quit smoking.** Nicotine is a highly addictive drug and cigarettes are very harmful to your health. The effects of tobacco are related to many illnesses that cause fatigue.
- **Fight insomnia.** Develop techniques and a sleep routine that will help you to rest fully and recuperate from tiredness.
- **Learn to relax.** There are many techniques, especially with complementary and natural therapies that can help you to relax and revitalize your energy. Developing personal relationships with friends and relatives can be helpful. Also, making time for gratifying activities and having fun is a great way to get over tiredness.

## NATURAL ALTERNATIVES

*With our stressful, busy lives, most of us experience tiredness sometimes. Daily commutes, overwork, straining physical exercise and changes in lifestyle can be treated, using effective, natural remedies:*

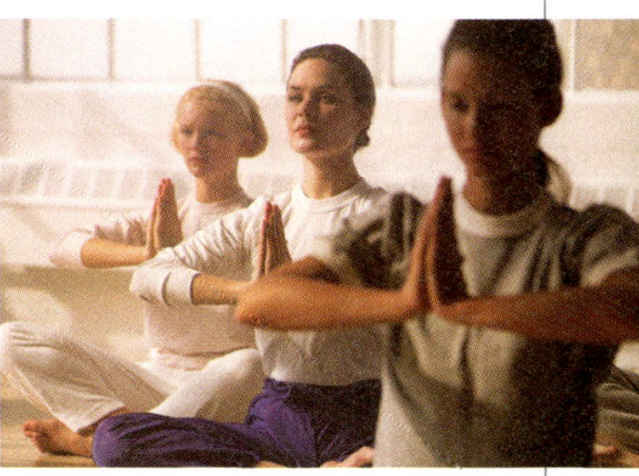

- ***Herbal medicine.*** *Revitalizing infusions, tinctures and teas.*
- ***Aromatherapy applications.*** *Using essential oils on the skin or during massages, or soaking in a hot bath with a few drops of an essential oil (see how to use aromatherapy to revitalize your energy in the list of* Essential oils from A to Z, *on page 47).*
- ***Eating energizing foods.*** *Among the basic foods, complex-carbohydrates found in wholegrain cereals are digested slowly, which permits sugar to be released into the bloodstream slowly. It is also good to eat bananas, apricots and almost all fruits that provide the body with necessary sugars. Beans as soy are a great way to incorporate low-fat protein into the diet (see* Foods to fight fatigue, *on page 56). However, it's good to consult your medical doctor before starting a new diet; and you should definitely seek medical advice if you suffer from diabetes or if you are overweight.*
- ***Alternative therapies.*** *To overcome tiredness there are techniques: yoga, meditation, reflexology, hydrotherapy, energizing* Chinese *self-massages –do-*in *and* qi gong*– (see* Complementary therapies, *from page 10).*

### SYMPTOMS OF NORMAL TIREDNESS

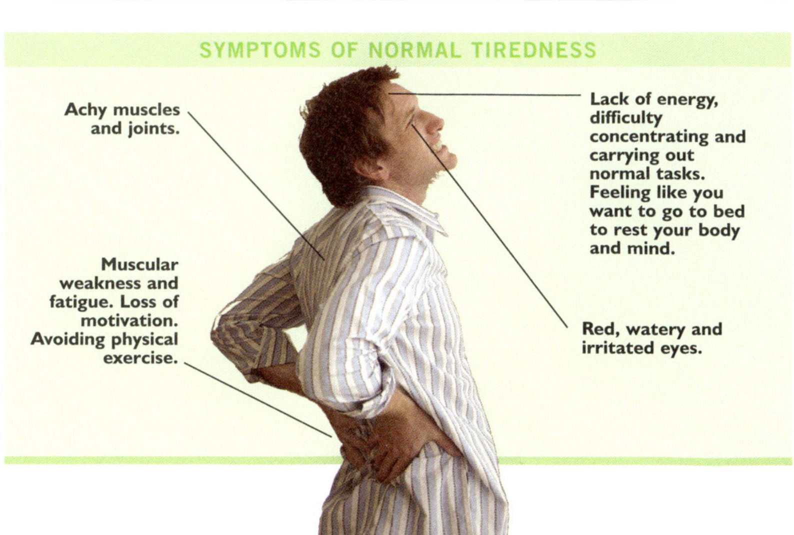

## CHANGE YOUR HABITS

If you are busy and constantly on the go, not exercising or taking out the time needed to rest completely can cause excessive tiredness. There are a number of solutions on hand to transform your home and office in sanctuaries for tranquility.

### At home

There are basic concepts based on the century old Chinese philosophy of *feng shui*, a way to mindfully organize your environment to bring harmony and restfulness into your life:

- Do not place your alarm clock, radios or stereos anywhere near the headboard of your bed or place where you rest. Also, avoid placing computers close to your legs. Electronic equipment have transformers that produce electromagnetic fields that when you are exposed to them over time can cause tiredness.
- Avoid cluttered areas, because they can pollute your vision and the lack of energy flow can affect the nervous system, alternating your vital energy flow.
- Don't combine contrasting colors (for example black and white) in the ceramic tile or flooring in the bathroom or kitchen because the contrast can cause visual fatigue.
- Keep your house dry and ventilated.

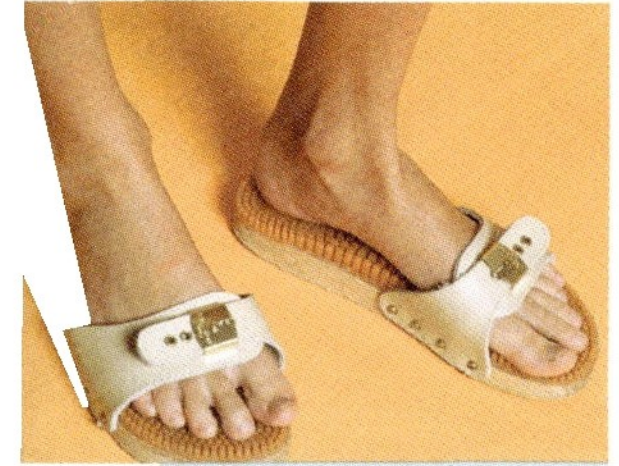

**SHOES**
**You should wear shoes for their utility not because they are in style. Narrow shoes, high heels and uncomfortable designs force the feet into positions that are unstable and unnatural, which not only exhaust your feet but your entire body.**

### In your free time

To help you rest up and energize it's good to go out, have fun and get away from your everyday responsibilities. Many entertaining and leisure activities can contribute to being able to rest. In addition, endorphins are released when you are having fun. Endorphins are chemicals produced in the brain in response to a variety of stimuli, they may be nature's cure for high levels of stress. They lead to feelings of euphoria, moderation of appetite, release of sex hormones and enhancement of the immune responses. Endorphins are released when you exercise, experience orgasms and laugh.

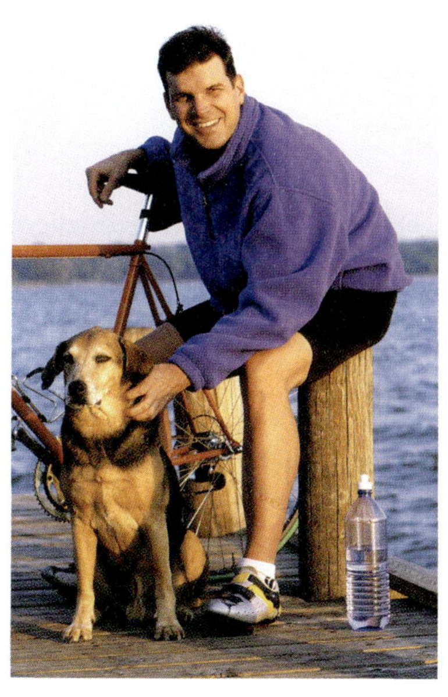

## At work

The clothes that you use during the day can also contribute to daily fatigue. To relieve tiredness –and other ailments– it's important to wear comfortable clothes; there is no reason to confuse formal wear with using uncomfortable clothes.

- For women, you should use the size of clothes that are best for your body, don't use tight clothes for fashion's sake. Tight clothes and uncomfortable fabrics can cause a sensation of exhaustion.
- For men, using a necktie too tight, constantly using a suit or using unnecessary jackets can add to tiredness during the day.
- Limit, if possible, the utilization of synthetic fabrics.

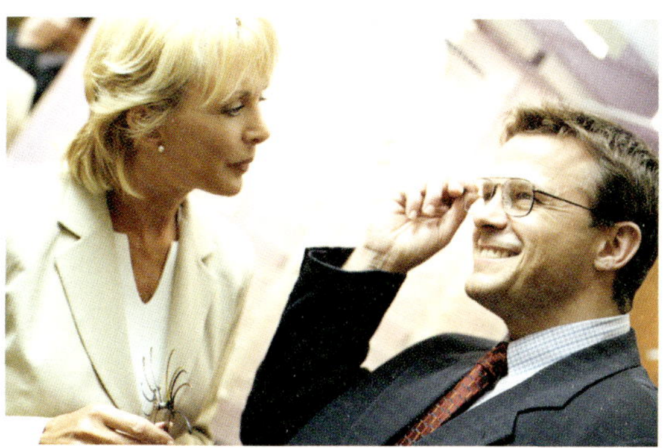

# Exercise and sports

A regular exercise program can help you to enjoy your body and to avoid tiredness caused by a sedentary lifestyle. It is important to choose physical activity that is appropriate for your age, sex and overall physical fitness, keeping in mind any illnesses or ailments.

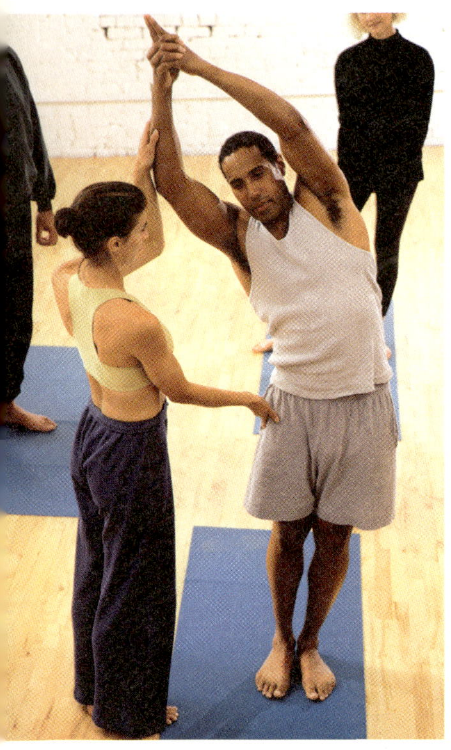

Not all physical exercises are the same, some may be better for a particular age group or for your overall fitness. It is recommended to consult your doctor before starting an exercise program to help you choose an activity which avoids overstraining or getting disappointed with your physical level. Studies have shown that regular exercise significantly increases life expectancy and improves overall health. An improved self-image and increased energy level are frequent added benefits of exercise.

Keeping your body in good working condition for daily life and health isn't about running marathons; it's about maintaining a healthy level of physical activity. You can start to exercise at any age, the young and old should incorporate regular physical activity into their everyday lives. Gradually building up the time spent doing the activity by adding a few minutes every few days, when your body feels stronger, faster and more flexible.

Choosing a fitness program can include a

variety of physical activities, from going to a gym, to playing a sport or walking daily. Aerobic activity is good for improving cardiovascular health, losing weight, toning the muscles and increasing your energy level. Aerobic activity is ideal for people who are recuperating from an ailment, who haven't exercised in a while, or for people who are over 50 years of age.

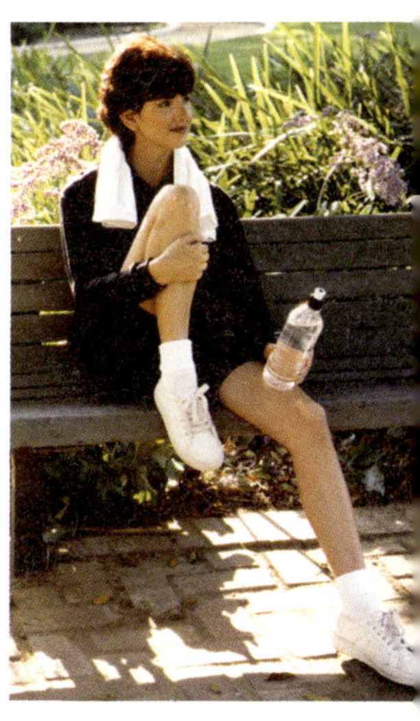

Competitive sports, have the same benefits as aerobic activity, but require time-commitment, a high-level of physical fitness and appropriate training to avoid injuries or other physical risks. It is recommended to begin an exercise program under the supervision of a physical trainer, and only after having a complete physical checkup.

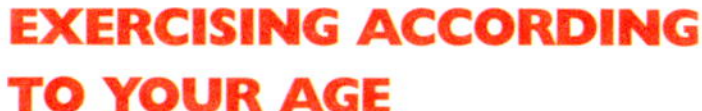

## EXERCISING ACCORDING TO YOUR AGE

**Between 18 and 35 years old**

This is one of the best stages in your life to practice sports, because your physical fitness is at its peak. It's ideal to practice sports during childhood because the benefits from physical activity later on in life will be greater. It's recommended to carry out a regular physical fitness routine so that your body stays toned and fit, increasing your stamina so that you don't get tired out as easily. If you exercise or train daily, it's advised to take a break at least one day a week, or to alternate between light exercise and intense physical training, so that your body doesn't get fatigued.

**Between 35 and 50 years old**

If you are in good health, you can do any

physical exercise or competitive sport, using precaution. Stamina, flexibility and strength begin to decrease during this age period, increasing the risk of injury and fatigue. It's best to work out at a moderate rate, three days a week. It's also recommended to practice activities that are beneficial for the health but low risk for injuries such as swimming, walking and biking. For those who have practiced sports or worked out regularly throughout life, you can train four to six days per week at a medium-high intensity. It's best to incorporate exercises that increase and support the body's stamina and flexibility, like running for 30 minutes or biking for an hour.

### Between 50 and 60 years old

Our bodies begin to change: we lose muscle mass, increase fat on the muscles and our capability to recuperate from tired muscles decreases. For this age group it is fundamental to keep active to stay as fit as possible.

Although it would be ideal to practice a competitive sport at this age, it is best advised to go to the gym or to go walking. If up to this age you haven't regularly exercised, it's best to start with a low-impact physical activity and to build up your resistance so that you get less tired. It is

**DAILY EXERCISE**

Many adults don't realize the amount of exercise that the body needs to stay healthy. It's important to keep in mind the benefits to help continue a regular exercise routine and avoid adapting to a sedentary lifestyle. However, in order to stay healthy, it is not necessary to exhaust your body doing rigorous exercises. Walking for half an hour or swimming 15 minutes a day is enough to keep our bodies healthy. Other day-to-day tasks such as washing the car, walking up stairs, going for a stroll (with a friend) and cleaning the house are all daily physical activities that keep up our physical stamina.

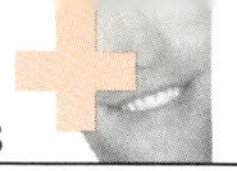

**SAFETY**

If you take a break from playing sports or working out because the body feels fatigued and after a period of rest you don't feel better, it is important to visit your doctor for a checkup. This prolonged tiredness can be a symptom of an illness or injury that can worsen by continued exercises or athletic training.

recommended to begin sports such as golf, swimming, walking or biking, always after consulting your physician. Symmetric sports are best, that's to say exercises that work out the left side of your muscle mass and the right side too, so that your entire body is equally strong. For those who have played sports or worked out throughout most of their lives, it's best to continue with the favorite sport, okayed by your doctor. However, alternate the sport with some type of gym work out that increases your flexibility like yoga, stretching or pilates.

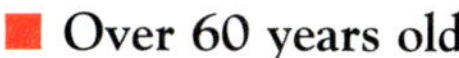

## Over 60 years old

Continued and controlled exercise increases the organs' resistance to aging and lowers muscular and cardiovascular deterioration. For those of us in this age group, an exercise routine can help to avoid a sedentary lifestyle and many illnesses. Recommended sports for this age group include swimming, aqua aerobics and walking.

**ATHLETE'S FATIGUE**

Among athletes, muscular and joint pains are frequent and common. Many times we ignore these pains until they begin to impede our normal daily activities. Sports injuries caused by fatigued muscles or joints are the most common among athletes. They can be prevented by stretching, warming up and correct training under a trainer's supervision. Loss of appetite, insomnia, irritability, decreased ability to recuperate and muscular or joint pains and cramps are symptoms of fatigue or over-training. In general, reducing intense physical exercise can reverse this situation to be able to return to normal physical activities.

# Yoga for fatigue

Yoga is a technique dating back thousands of years, its philosophical principles and techniques are based on creating harmony between mind, body and spirit. Regularly practicing yoga *asanas* or poses relaxes the body while at the same time revitalizes the lack of energy which causes you to be tired.

Tiredness is a symptom of an imbalance of strength and energy that yoga can help to put back into harmony. While many *asanas* require your body to work hard, over time you will benefit from yoga's relaxing effects: correct breathing, improved oxygen flow in the body, increased energy and better blood circulation.

It's best to practice yoga for 20 minutes, on a padded mat, in the morning before starting your day or in the evening at the end of your day.

It's also advised to begin these exercises with an instructor who can help to familiarize you with the techniques.

**GENTLE EXERCISE**

**Yoga is a discipline designed to improve your flexibility and harmony. The exercises use gentle movements without straining your body. When practicing the *asanas* remember not to strain yourself. There is no need to push yourself too far. Remember to use gentle movements and don't push your body into a pose. Throughout time and willpower, you will improve your body's health naturally and get in tune with your body. It is important to remember to use your body with moderation, patience and consistency to prevent side effects like sore muscles or tiredness.**

## GETTING PREPARED

As with all exercises, before practicing yoga postures or *asanas*, you should prepare your body through a series of stretching exercises to warm up your muscles and to release tension.

### Rocking chair

This pose is good for loosening and toning your muscles. It is used as a series of movements practiced at the beginning of a yoga session, although it is also good to practice this pose at the end of a session, before meditation. As the name suggests, this *asana* rocks the body, while at the same time increasing your muscle flexibility, releasing tensions, energizing and improving the flow of energy in the spinal cord. It's best to use a moderate rhythm, inhaling through the nose when you move backward and exhaling through the mouth when you move forward.

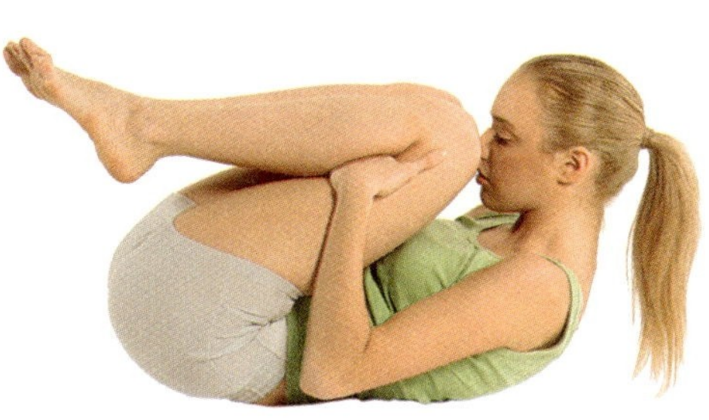

***1.*** *Sit on the floor, with your chin pressed against your chest. Bend your legs, with your feet pressed against the floor. Place your hands behind your knees, with your thumbs pointed outward. Keep your chin pressed to your chest to prevent back injuries.*

***2.*** *Lift up your feet, supporting them with your arms. Inhale and bring the body backward, maintaining the position of your legs and chin. Rock back and forth five or six times, keeping the legs bent to get the body ready.*

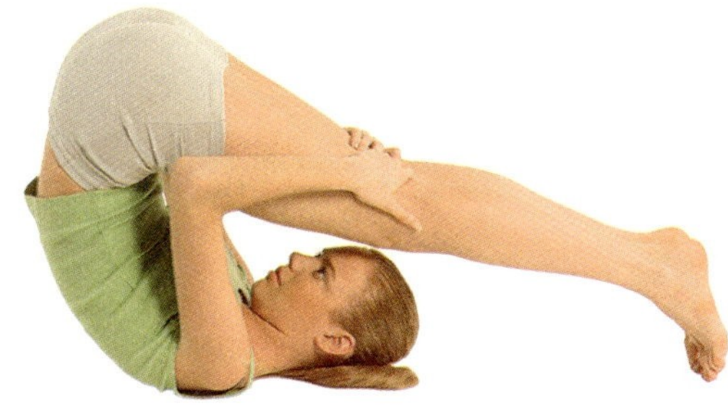

***3.*** *Once the body has enough elasticity, use the motion to bring the torso backward and to stretch back your legs behind your head. If you can, try to touch the floor with the tips of your toes. Exhale and rock forward, without lifting up your chin. Repeat seven or eight times without stopping. Next, lie back down for a minute or two to relax your body.*

## BREATHING FOR RELAXATION

Breathing is the body's most important function, which provides the primary element that our bodies need: oxygen. Yoga uses a number of techniques that concentrate on breathing, making yoga ideal for oxygenating, revitalizing and fighting against tiredness.

Nasal breathing –naturally practiced since birth– carries a connection to the cosmic Universe's rhythm. As we grow up and our natural biological processes accelerate, our synchronism with the Universe alters, giving way to a daily vertigo. When we breathe through our mouths, we absorb more air in less time, but without filling our lungs. Also, when we exhale we don't expel all the carbon dioxide from our lungs.

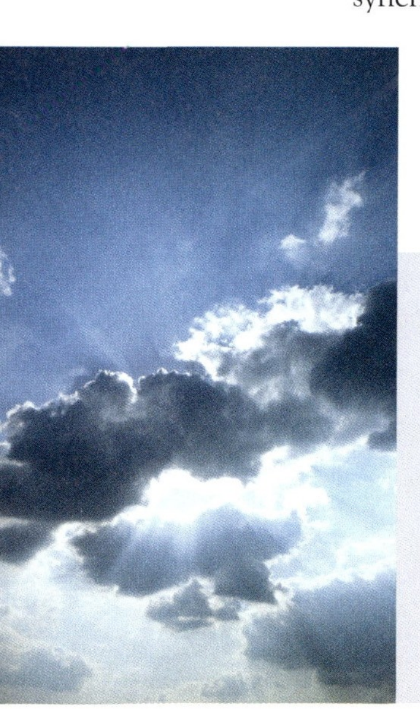

**COSMIC BREATHING**

**Even though breathing is an instinctive biological function, we tend to breathe incorrectly. The most natural canal for the breath is the nose:**

- **The tiny hairs inside the nostril filter and purify the air.**
- **The air is warmed by contact with the veins inside the nostrils.**
- **It relaxes the nervous system.**
- **It purifies the body by expelling carbon dioxide.**

## BREATHING TO RELAX

We have put together a list of exercises that will help you to breathe consciously, to energize you and to revitalize your body, especially when you are tired. However, you should take note that sometimes these exercises can make you dizzy. If this happens, it's best to take a break from the exercises and practice them later with less intensity.

## Abdominal and Diaphragmatic Breathing

Diaphragmatic breathing uses the diaphragm, a muscle located under our ribs and above our stomach. When we breathe in, we push the muscle down and our stomach moves forward. When we breathe out, the diaphragm moves back to resting position and the abdomen moves back in. It's best to do this breathing technique lying down, on the floor or on a padded mat.

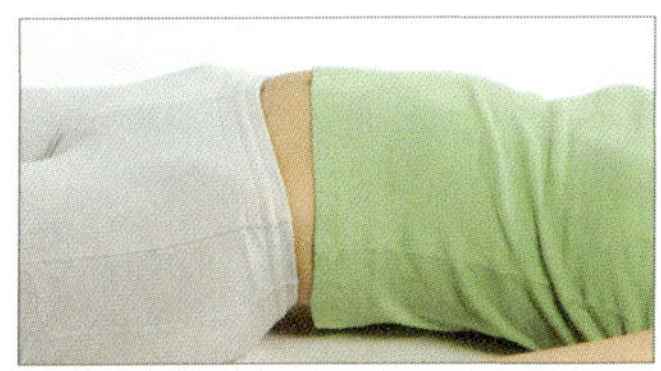

*1. Take a deep breath, inhaling slowly through your nose and expanding your abdomen. Concentrate on your energy in that spot.*

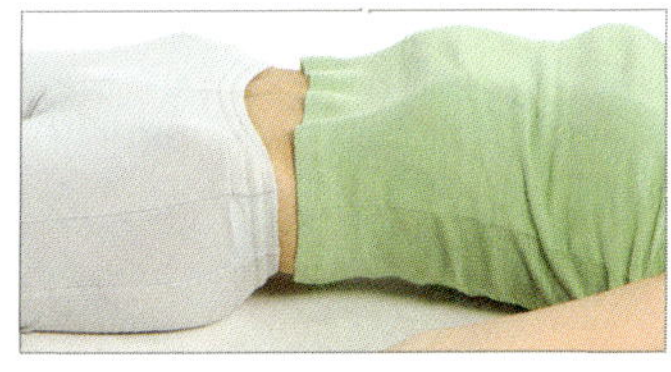

*2. Slowly exhale, contracting your abdomen before taking another breath. While exhaling, when the air passes through the throat make a sound as if you were snoring. Repeat 4 or 5 complete breaths.*

## Alternate breathing

This exercise consists of inhaling and exhaling through the nostrils alternately. Use your right hand, place your index and middle fingers below your eyebrow and use your thumb to close one nostril at a time, alternating between the right and left nostril.

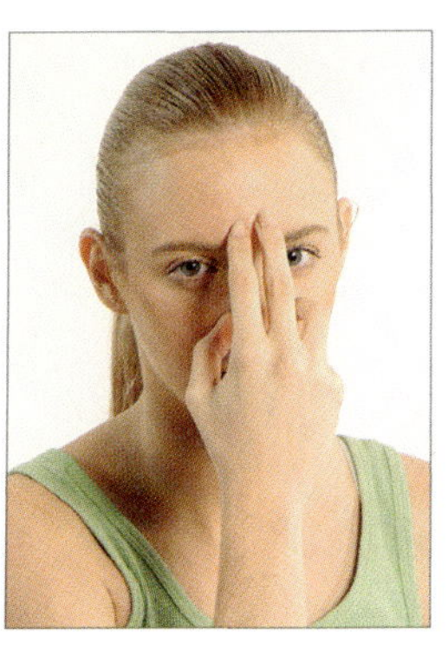

*1. Sit with your back straight and your head slightly tilted downward. Begin to exhale through your left nostril, while you close your right nostril with your thumb. Inhale through the same nostril.*

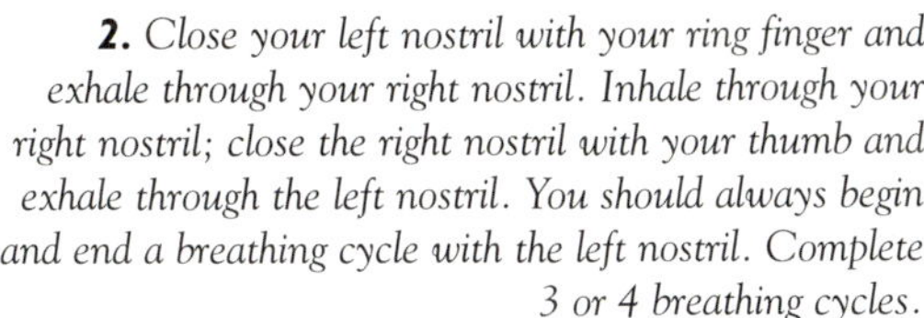

*2. Close your left nostril with your ring finger and exhale through your right nostril. Inhale through your right nostril; close the right nostril with your thumb and exhale through the left nostril. You should always begin and end a breathing cycle with the left nostril. Complete 3 or 4 breathing cycles.*

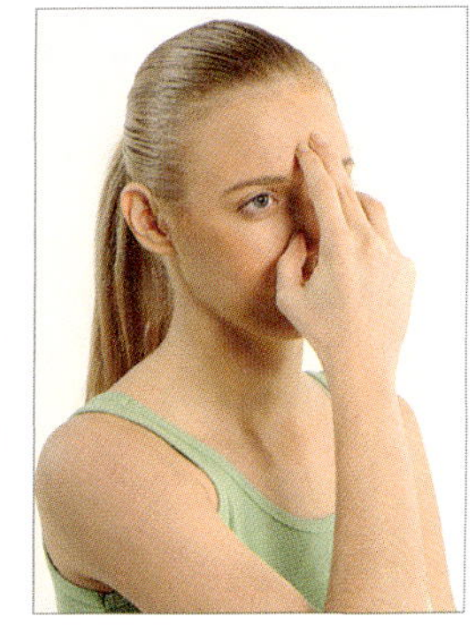

## POSTURES TO RELIEVE YOUR TENSION

When you are suffering from tiredness, nothing is better to energize the body than yoga. *Asanas* also bring a total state of relaxation.

### The Seated forward bend

This *asana* uses slow movements, and is an ideal exercise for moments when you feel exhausted. It brings vitality, literally stretches the back part of the body, at the same time stretches the vertebrae and stimulates blood flow of the back. This pose clears your mind and calms the spirit.

**1.** *Begin by sitting, with your legs together and stretched forward. Keep you back straight and your arms on the sides of your body, supported by your palms. Your body should form a 90 degree angle. Take in a deep breath through the nose and stretch your arms above your head as high as you can, stretching the spine. Do not arch the back.*

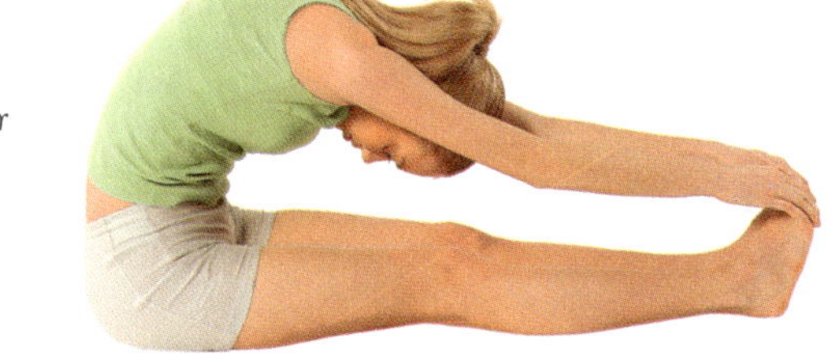

**2.** *As you exhale bring your chest toward your thighs. Bring your hands to your feet and, if you can, wrap your fingers around them. Breathe comfortably, while you exhale lowering your torso as far as you can. It's ideal to bring your abdomen to your thighs. The idea is to continue right down and hold on to whichever part of your legs or feet you can comfortably reach. You can also place a cord behind your feet and grab onto it instead of your toes.*

## Reverse pose

This exercise helps the body to recuperate, to clear and calm an exhausted mind and to relieve headaches. It also helps to improve blood circulation especially for the blood flow to the brain.

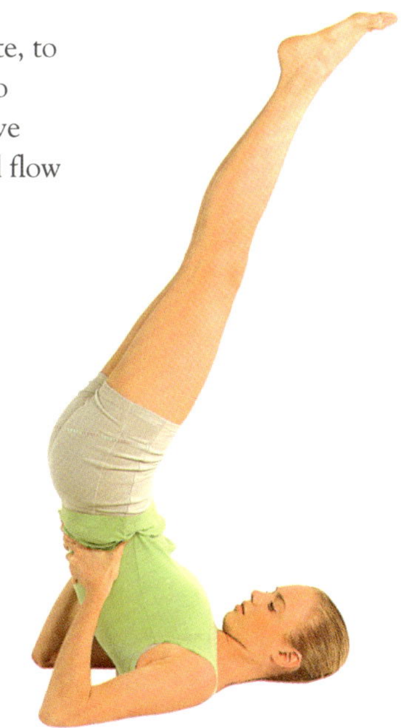

*Begin by lying down with the palms of your hands on the floor, your legs together and looking forward. Lift up your legs and then your torso. Support your waist with your hands, so that your legs and torso are at an angle. Your feet should be raised directly above your head. Stay in this position for as long as you feel comfortable, breathing slowly. Next, slowly lower the legs and relax your body for a few moments.*

## Relaxing pose

Although this is a passive pose, this *asana* is beneficial for its ability to relieve tensions and energize the body. Dedicating 10 minutes to this *asana* is equivalent to two hours of deep sleep because of its capacity to recover mental and physical vital energy.

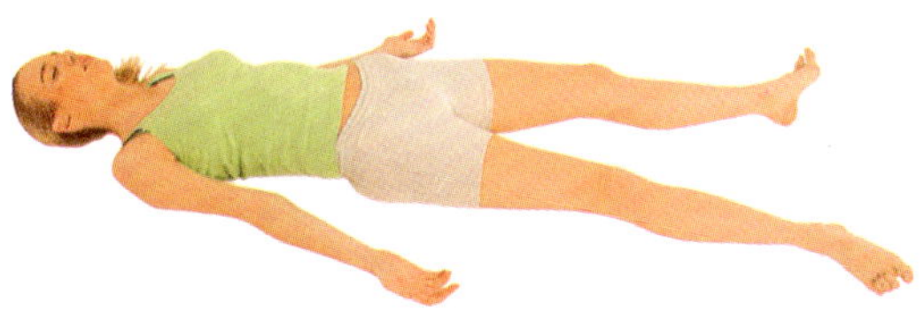

*Lie on your back looking for the most comfortable position for your body: shoulders relaxed, back straight, loose hips and legs slightly apart. The tips of your toes should face outward; your arms, a bit separated from the body, with the palms of your hands open and facing upward. Close your eyes, breathing slowly and deeply. Concentrate on tensing and relaxing each muscle, from your toes to your head. You will feel the weight of your body. Stay in this position for a few minutes, with your eyes closed and without breathing deeply. You will rest significantly in a brief amount of time.*

## MUDRAS FOR FATIGUE

This technique, dating back thousands of years, uses *mudras* or physical gestures considered sacred for their energetic power to relieve tiredness. Practicing *mudras* is easy and doesn't require a professional practitioner or instructor.

There are four *mudras* or gestures to treat problems of fatigue. You may practice these gestures three times a day for 15 minutes. You can practice *mudras* in any place (except for the dawn *mudra*). Over time and with constant practice you will recuperate lost energy.

### Dawn mudra

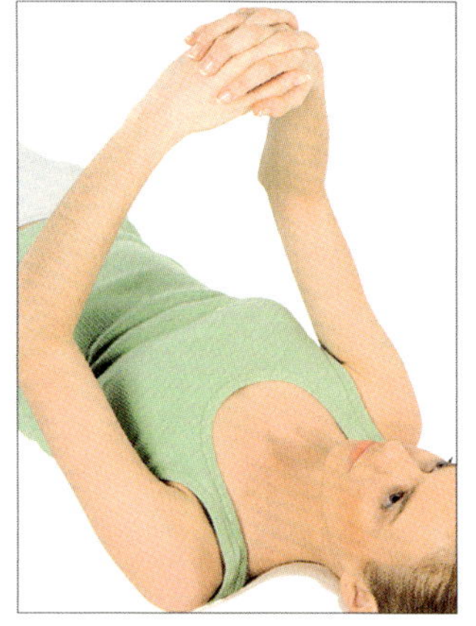

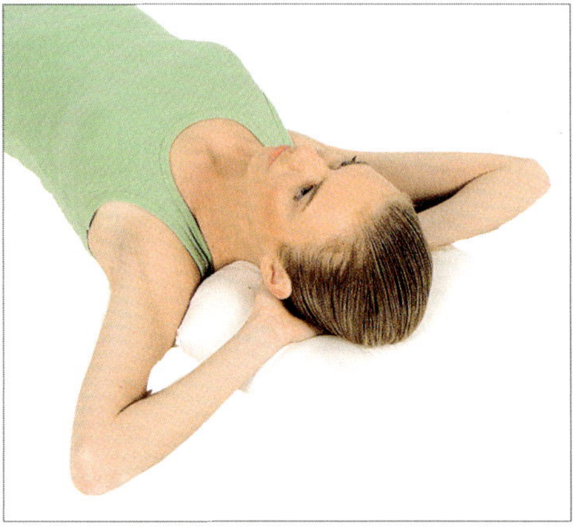

**1.** *In the morning, before getting out of bed, clasp your fingers so that your right thumb sits on your left thumb and gently press.*

**2.** *Next, bring your hands behind your head and breathe deeply several times, while you open your eyes and mouth. Press your elbows backward against your pillow. You will feel a wave of energy that will help you face the day with more strength.*

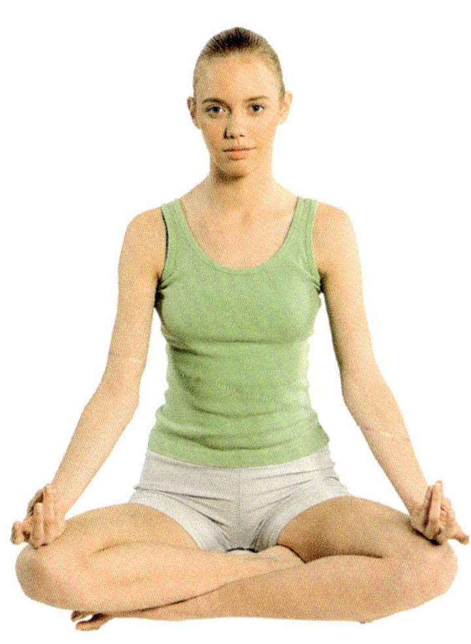

## Earth mudra

*With your palms facing upward, place the point of your thumbs at the base of your ring fingers. Apply gentle pressure while the rest of the fingers are stretched out. Repeat with both hands. The ring finger symbolizes the earth element, which is stimulated to recuperate strength and physical and mental stamina. You can practice this* mudra *in the Lotus position or any other position or place.*

## Sky mudra

*With your palms facing upward and your thumbs and middle fingers pressed together. Keep the rest of your fingers extended. Practice this* mudra *with both hands. This gesture stimulates optimism and a good mood. As with the earth* mudra, *it can be practiced in the Lotus or any other position, without necessarily being an* asana.

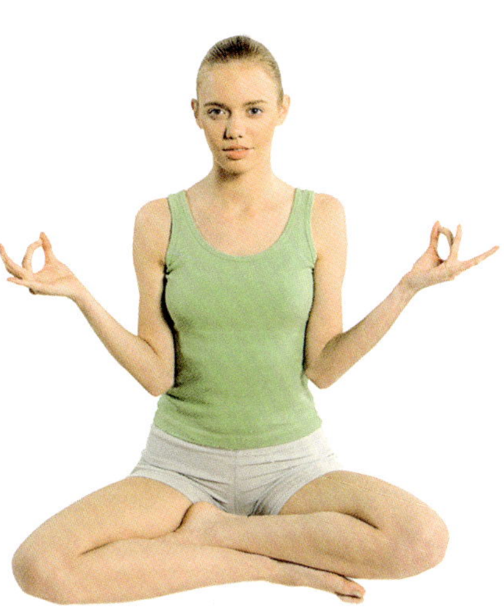

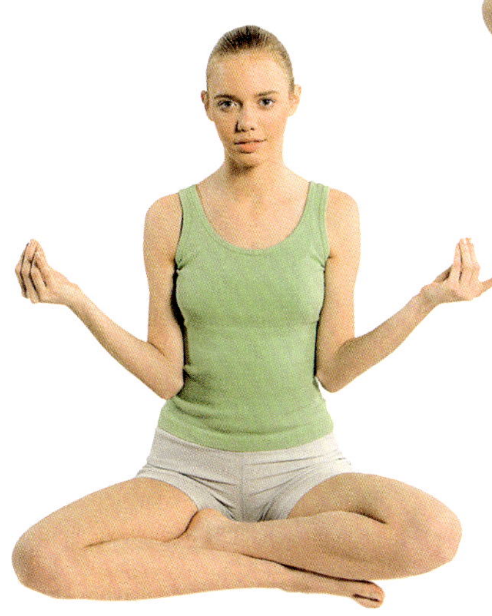

## Purifying mudra

*With the palm of your left hand facing upward with your thumb, middle, ring and pinkie finger pressed together. Your index finger should be extended, as if you were pointing to something. Repeat on your right hand but this time press your thumb, index, middle and ring fingers together and point with your pinkie. This* mudra *detoxifies your body and mind. This* mudra *can be practiced in the Lotus position or any other position.*

# Restful massages

This series of massages is great to help you relax and to fight stress. They can be done in your own home with the assistance of a relative.

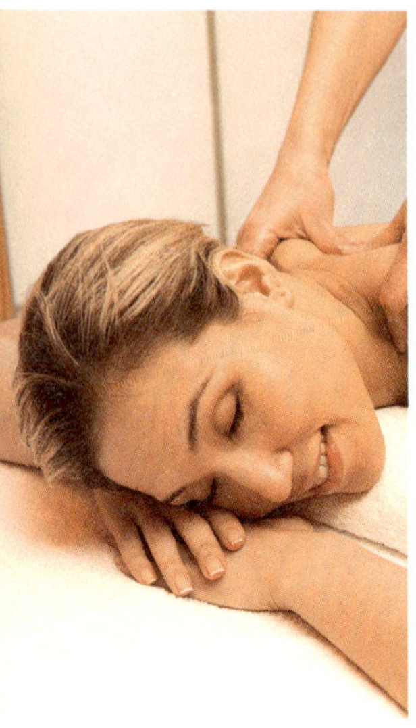

For massages to be truly therapeutic, there are certain guidelines to follow when giving a massage or doing a self-massage. Here are a few tips:

- Pick a quiet and warm room with plenty of light and ventilation.
- The session should be done in silence or with soft music in the background.
- The surface on which the person receiving the massage is lying shouldn't be soft.
- When you are receiving a massage it's good to empty your mind, to help relaxation.

## TENSION RELIEVING MASSAGE

This is a series of massages to stimulate blood and lymphatic flow, raising your energy. They help to relieve headaches and sore muscles, in addition to leaving a sense of total well-being. It's recommended to do these massages as a complete series to give truly therapeutic results.

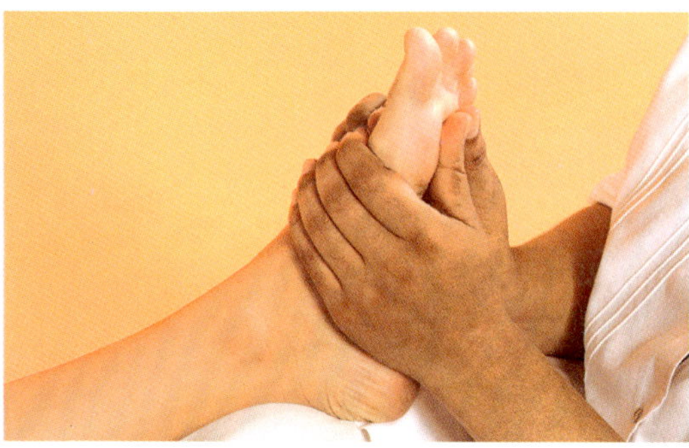

*1. Begin with the foot, sliding your thumbs down the foot. This not only relaxes the feet, but the entire body.*

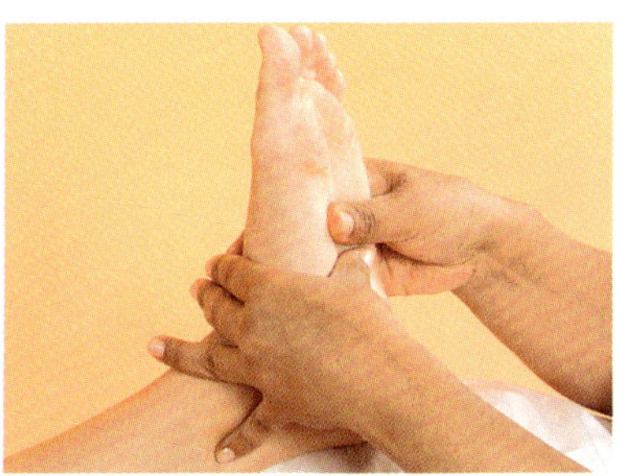

**2.** *Stimulate the central part of the foot, using pressure in different areas where you accumulate tension. This exercise stimulates blood flow.*

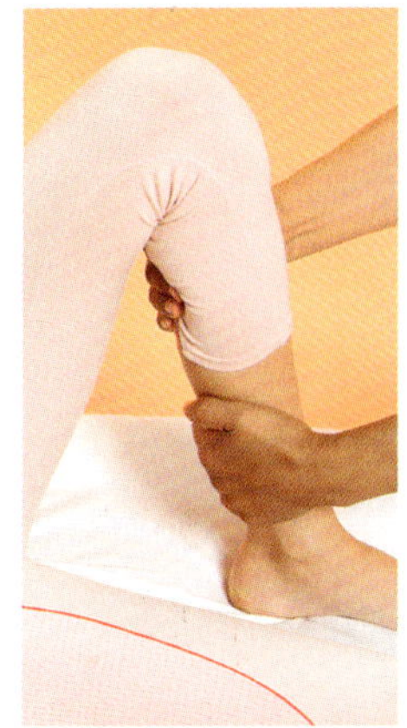

**3.** *Massage the calf muscle to relax tension and to increase blood circulation in the legs.*

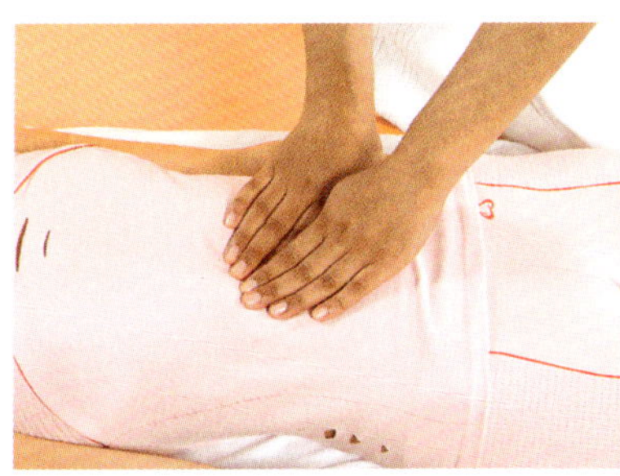

**4.** *Work on the abdomen using circular massages. This massage connects, distends and restores energy in the center of the body.*

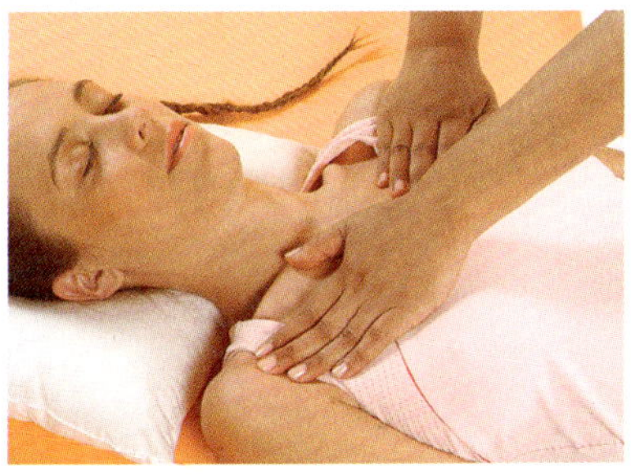

**5.** *Press your hands gently on the recipient's shoulders to release negative energy in the area near the heart. This pression opens the arteries and activates cardiac rhythm.*

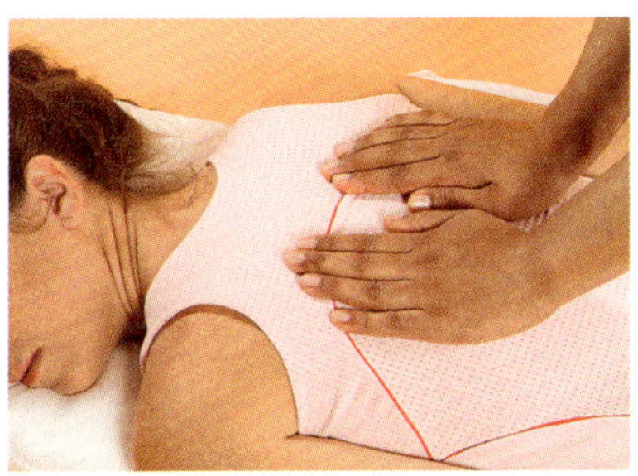

**6.** *Place your hands on the back, the area where we most store tensions. This helps to release blocked energy from the spinal column.*

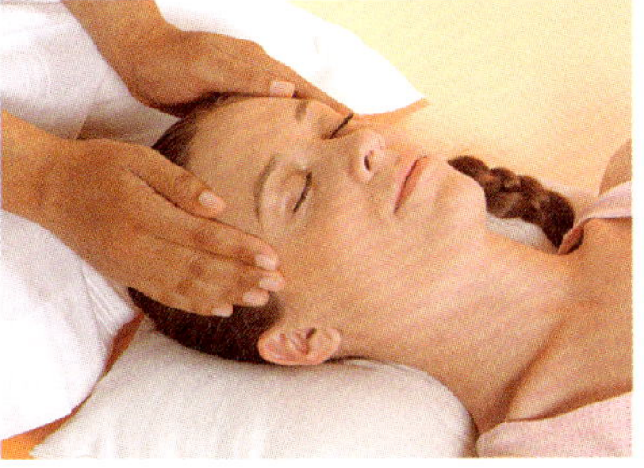

**7.** *Massage the temples to relax better. This movement helps to clear the mind and release worries.*

# Revitalizing self-massages

This is a series of simple and efficient techniques to give you a "pick-me-up", which will energize and invigorate your body.

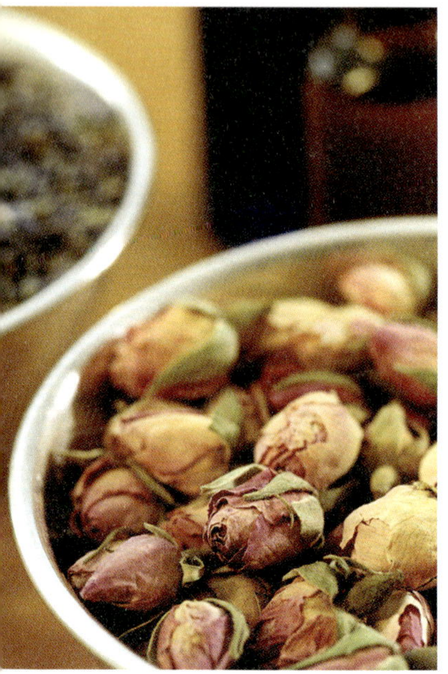

This massage can be done at any time of the day you have to take a rest, in private and after taking a hot bath. For this massage to be more effective you should prepare an appropriate atmosphere before giving yourself a self-massage: warm room, soft lighting, and inviting colors. More important than the time you can dedicate to the massage, it's best to choose a moment when you won't be interrupted. The following massages are based on *shiatsu*, an Eastern technique that uses finger pressure on determined points to recover and balance the body's energy.

*1. To restore vital energy. Wrap your hand around your foot and keep firm pressure. Gently hit the base of the foot with the edge of the palm of your hand.*

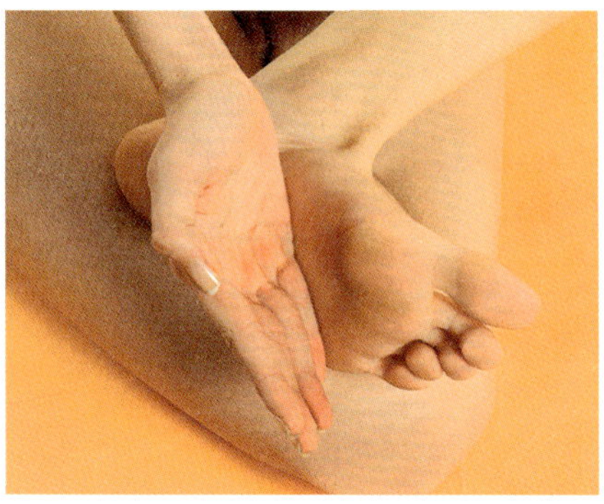

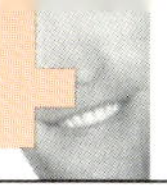

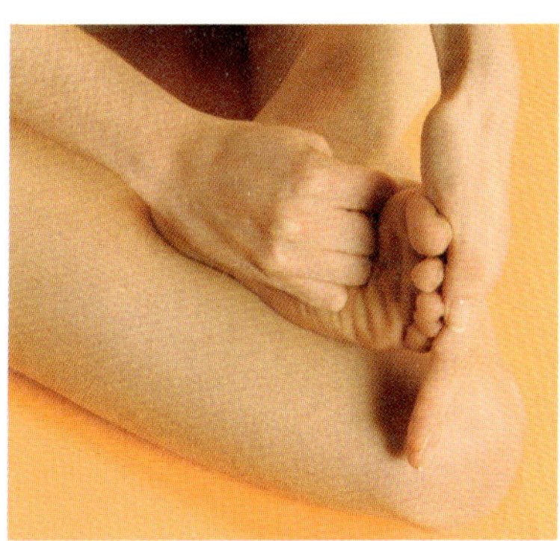

**2.** *To relieve tension. Wrap your hand around your foot and with the other make a fist and rub your foot with your knuckles, using circular movements.*

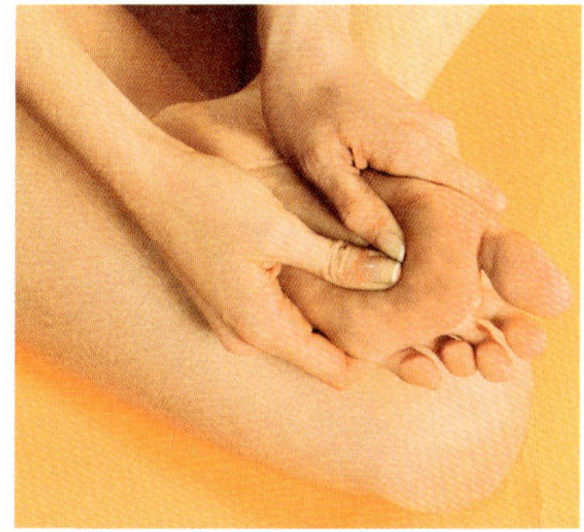

**3.** *To relieve anxiety. Place the thumb of one hand next to the thumb of the other and gently press on the center of the base of the foot. Keep breathing deeply.*

## AREAS TO WORK ON TO RELIEVE FATIGUE

**On the legs.** This point is located the width of your hand below your inner knee joint, in the hollow point between the femur and the muscle. Press on this point on both legs to relieve pains, especially from the waist down.

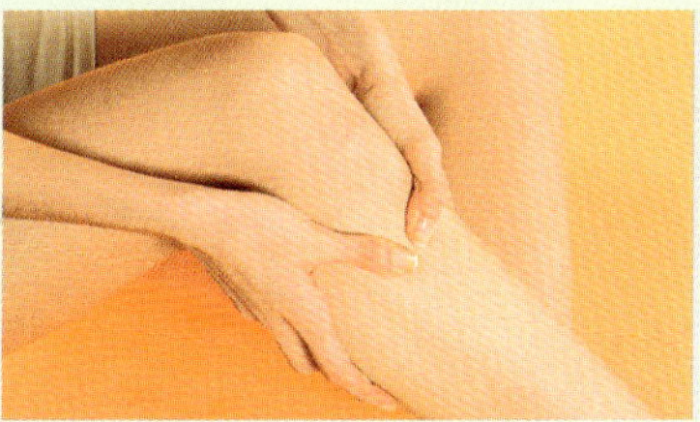

**On the shoulders.** Lift up your arm and look for the hollow place below the shoulder muscle. Once you've located the point apply pressure with your index fingers and thumbs; lower your arm and begin to massage by applying even pressure. Repeat on your other shoulder.

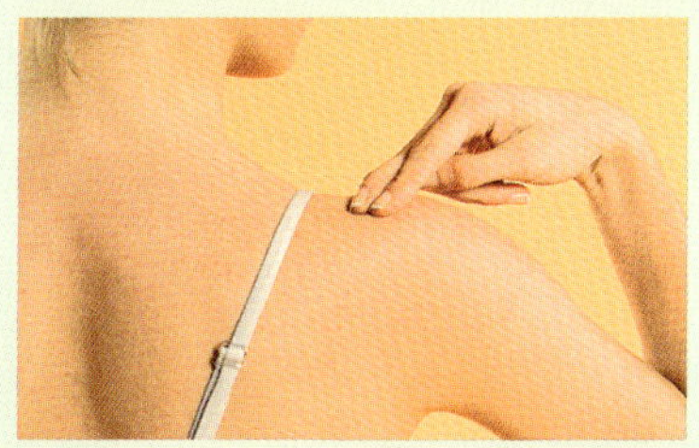

**On the wrists.** This point is found on the inner part of each of the wrists. Rub with your thumbs. Press on each wrist to relieve physical fatigue. This technique helps to relieve intense exhaustion.

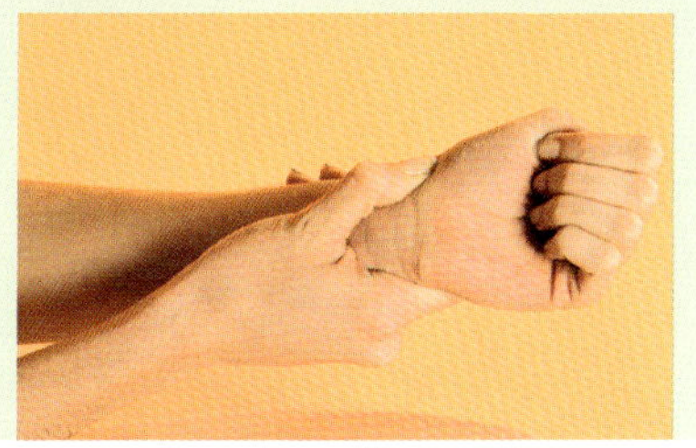

# Qi gong energy exercise

*Qi gong* self-massage originates in Chinese medicine, it is a series of techniques for stimulating and balancing the flow of *chi* energy with soft movements that harmonize the body's functions.

During the practice of *qi gong*, the hands are transmitters and receptors of energy. The technique trains the hands to become sensitive and efficient in detecting energy channels and the *laogong* point and a key tool called the Sword.

**The center of the palm of your hand is where the *laogong* is found, where a number of meridian channels meet. When you are giving a *qi gong* massage or self-massage, keep in mind that this point is a radar for detecting blocks, energy sources and deficiencies.**

When beginning *qi gong* massages it is important to clear your mind and concentrate on your hands and the part you are massaging. For more stimulating effects, repeat the massages between 15 and 30 times or for 10 minutes.

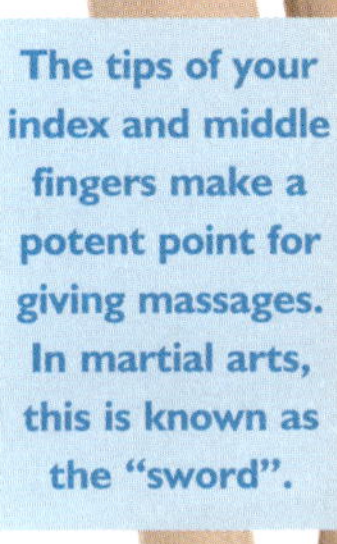

**The tips of your index and middle fingers make a potent point for giving massages. In martial arts, this is known as the "sword".**

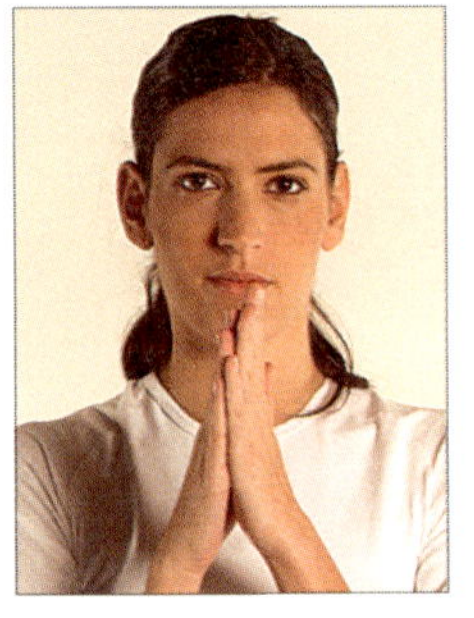

**Friction on the hands.** *Before beginning a* qi gong *session and between massages it is important to rub the palms of your hands together. During this technique you should concentrate on the* laogong *point and the points on the fingers.*

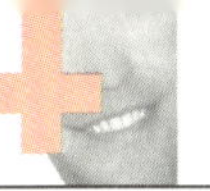

## REACTIVATING THE CHI

To use the *qi gong* self-massages, stand up with your body relaxed and your feet about shoulder width apart. This technique will activate your vital energy.

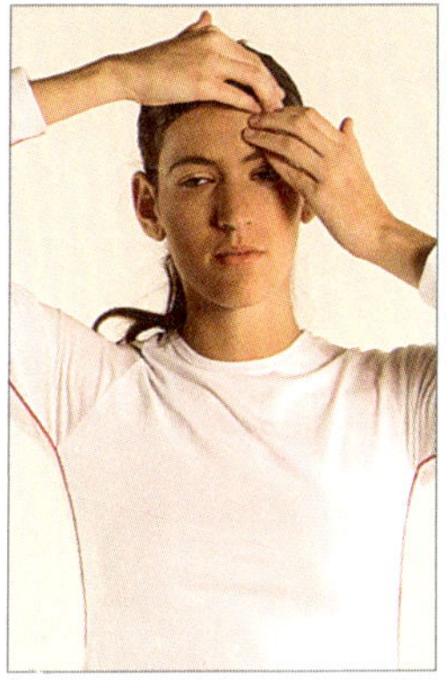

**On the forehead.** *Massage your forehead with one hand and then the other, rubbing from one temple to the other. This technique activates the nervous system and the blood flow in this sensitive area of the head.*

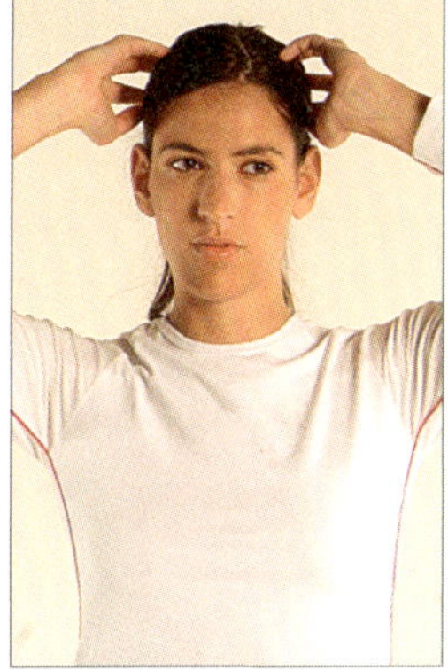

**On the scalp.** *Place your fingertips on your scalp, on the sides of your head. Rub forward and then backward. Next, apply pressure with your nails, as if they were a comb and use friction in the same way. This massage helps to stimulate your vital energy and fight against fatigue.*

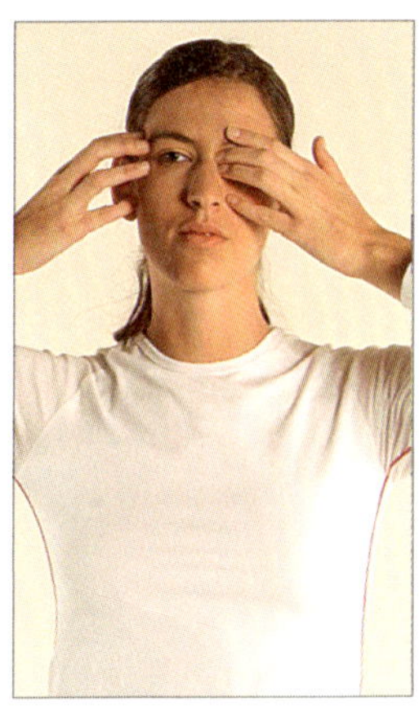

**On the eyes.** *Cup your hands. Place your index and your pinkie over your eye sockets, while your other two fingers touch your eyelids lightly. The massage consists of an energetic friction from the eyes to the temples. This helps your eyes take a rest.*

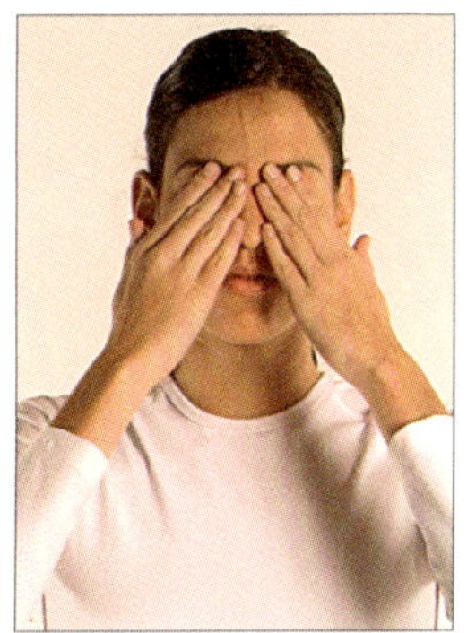

**On the face.** *Place your hands in front of your face. Rub down, starting with your forehead, in front of your eyes, until your chin. Separate your hands and apply friction, moving upward. This technique invigorates the energy in the face, tones the skin and facial muscles, preventing premature wrinkles.*

**On the ming men.** This center is an important place in the body, where our vital energy is stored. It is located between the second and third lumbar vertebrae, just beneath the two kidneys.
This self-massage is practiced in two steps, benefitting the flow of energy through the meridians and harmonizing the function of the kidneys. Make a fist, making sure that your thumb sits on your index finger, forming a circle. Keep your wrist lose. This posture is called the Tiger's mouth.

**1.** *With your fists rub the* ming men *point, using circular motions, 15 times clock-wise and 15 times counter clock-wise.*

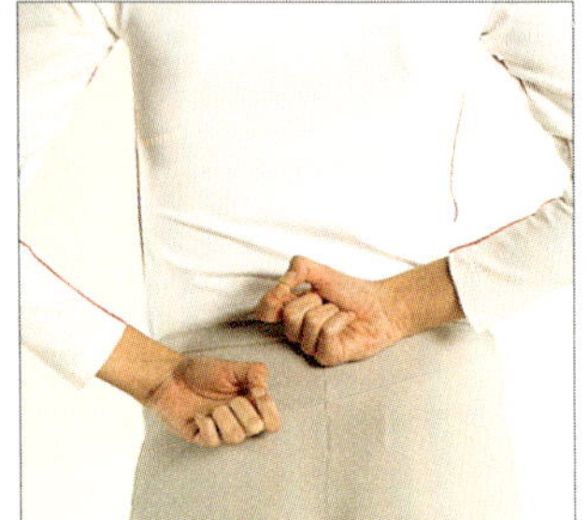

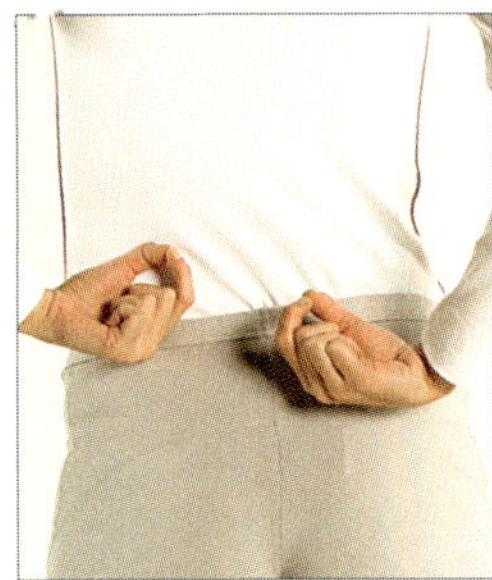

**2.** *Next, with your fists gently tap on the ming men points, alternating between the right and left hand side.*

**On the arms.** This massage is used to activate the flow of the *chi* (vital energy) through the meridian acupuncture points in the arms.

**1.** *With your left hand open, massage the right arm, first on the inside of the arm to the shoulder with your fingertips.*

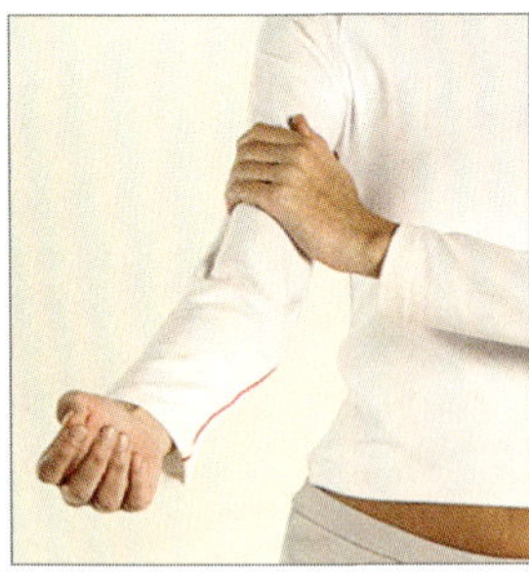

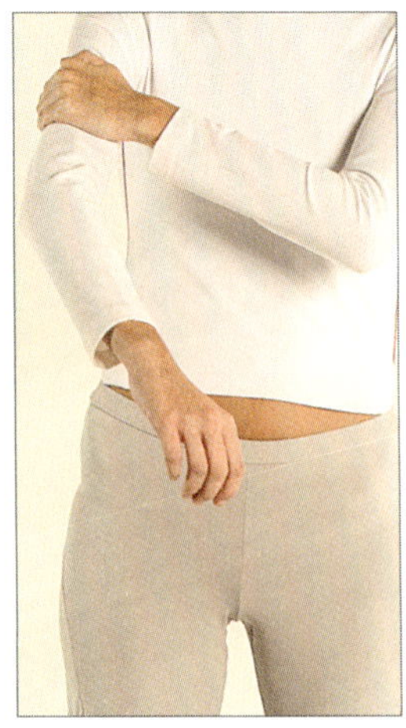

**2.** *Next, massage up the outer arm until you reach the shoulder. Repeat 15 times and change arms.*

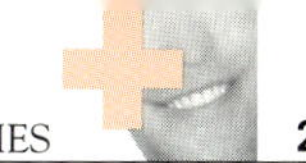

**On the dantian.** The *dantian* refers to the central point in the lower abdomen, three fingers beneath the navel where the vital energy is refined and converted into subtle energy for distribution to the rest of the organism. This massage will make you feel as if you have heat running through the abdominal cavity. This self-massage is practiced in two stages.

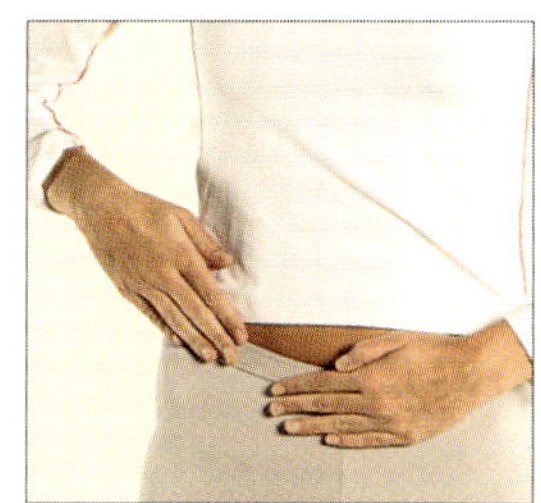

*1. First, place your hands over the point and diagonally rub 30 times, with one hand moving upward and the other downward.*

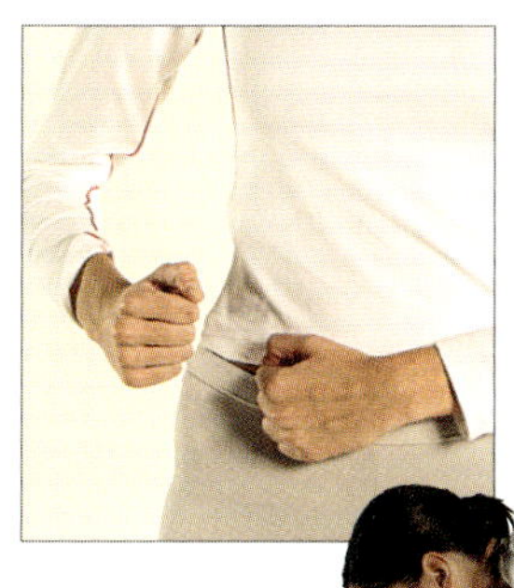

*2. Next, place your hands in the "tiger's mouth" position and gently tap on the* dantian *30 times, to distribute energy.*

**On the arms.** This technique stimulates the circulation of the *chi* through the meridians in the legs. The same friction technique is used on the arms and the legs.

*With the palms of your hands massage the outer thigh, until your ankle. Next, massage up the inner part of the legs, until the thigh and then massage downward. Repeat 30 times.*

## AN ENERGIZING EXERCISE

**This massage helps when you are exhausted, improves concentration and relieves headaches.**

1. **Begin standing with your legs parallel shoulder width apart and your knees slightly bent. Your arms should stay at the sides of your body; your shoulders relaxed.**
2. **Lift up you arms, straighten with the palms facing upward, to the height of your shoulders. Whilst, breathing deeply, direct the breath toward the *dantian*, as if gathering the energy that is generated from there.**
3. **Next, inhale and bend your forearms placing your hands on your shoulders. Exhale while you release from this position.**

# Resting your feet

Reflexology is a natural healing art based on the study and practice of the principle that there are reflexes in the body –especially on the hands and feet– that correspond to the body's organs and glands. Applying stimulation and pressure to the feet or hands has a similar effect to a total body massage.

Daily activity and excessive physical work over short periods of time can exhaust your body, bringing on bouts of fatigue. Reflexology or reflexotherapy releases blocked energy and helps it flow. There are connections between different parts of the body. Reflexology is not an exact science, but is considered a natural healing art.

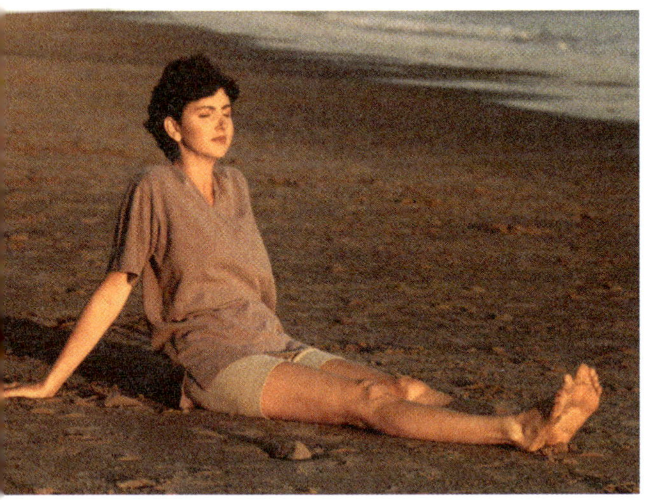

Reflexology has been used since around 3,000 B.C. particularly in China, but also in Malaysia and India. However, archeologists have found paintings referring to this technique in the Egyptian pyramids. Modern reflexology is based on the work of US physician William H. Fitzgerald, who in the early 20th century developed the ancient Oriental healing art of using pressure to relieve pains into a usable diagnostic therapy. Fitzgerald's nurses aid, Eunice Ingham, further pioneered a reflexology foot chart, which we use as a guide today and have included on this page.

## FOOT REFLEXOLOGY

There are a number of reflexology zones on the body, including the hands and ears. However, the foot is the area with most concentrated energy pathways and the easiest and most effective technique to practice. We've put together a beginners guide to foot reflexology. The essential points to treat tiredness are drawn in the diagram:

- On both feet: the areas representing the neck, shoulders, waist, spinal column, sacrum, coccyx, solar plexus, head and heart.
- On the outer part of the feet: lower back, knee, leg and back.
- On the inner part of the foot: the sacral, lumbar, thoracic and cervical areas. And on the instep, the hip.

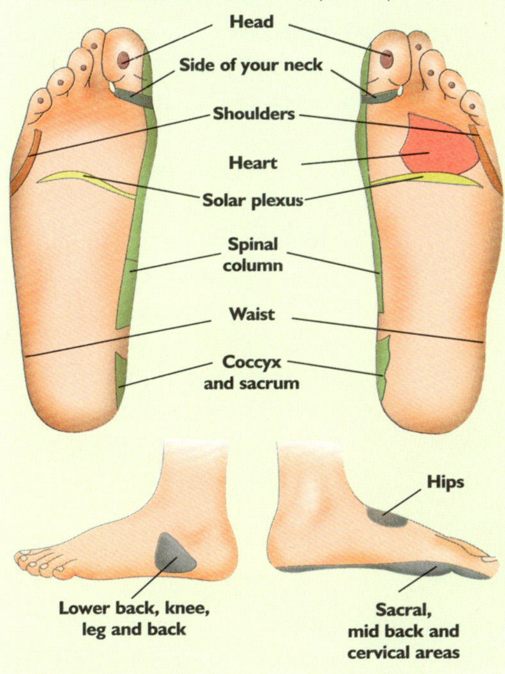


### STIMULATING DETAILS

- For tiredness a reflexology massage can be used to revitalize you at any time. However, the best time of the day to practice reflexology is in the morning because it prepares your body to start the day and to face everyday stress and taxing tasks. It can also be good to practice in the afternoon to decongest and relieve tension.
- It's always best to use high quality essential oils and foot creams.
- You can light incense sticks and put on soft music: taking care where you apply reflexology is a good way to improve results.
- Don't forget to take time for a foot massage for the health of the entire body.

## FOR PERSONAL RELAXATION

Reflexology, is based on the study of meridians that run throughout the whole body. Although an experienced practitioner should apply reflexology, there are massages based on this technique that you can do yourself to relieve discomfort. There are a number of techniques to treat tiredness, which activate lost or blocked vital energy.

### Getting ready

Before giving yourself a reflexology massage, it's recommended to sit in a comfortable position so that you can reach your feet. Do not bend your back, because you will block the flow of your breath. Although you can give yourself a massage with your socks on, it's best to do these exercises in your bare feet. Begin with a relaxing manual technique: wrap your hand around your ankle and roll your foot with your other hand.

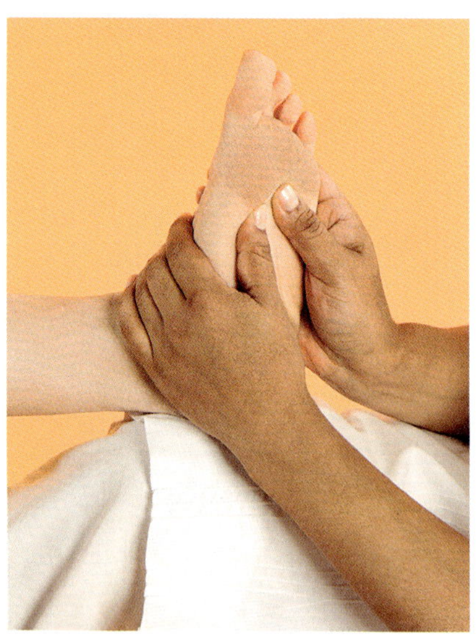

### Self-massages that relieve

After getting ready and following the diagram with the reflex points in the feet (see *Foot Reflexology* box, on page 31), you can begin with the following exercises when you feel tired and to give you a pick-me-up.

*1. Begin by applying pressure to the central point in the left foot to release built up tension. This point corresponds to the heart, an area where excess tension tends to be stored.*

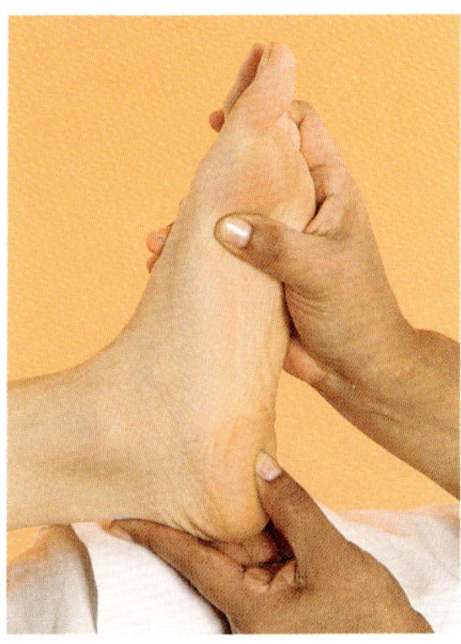

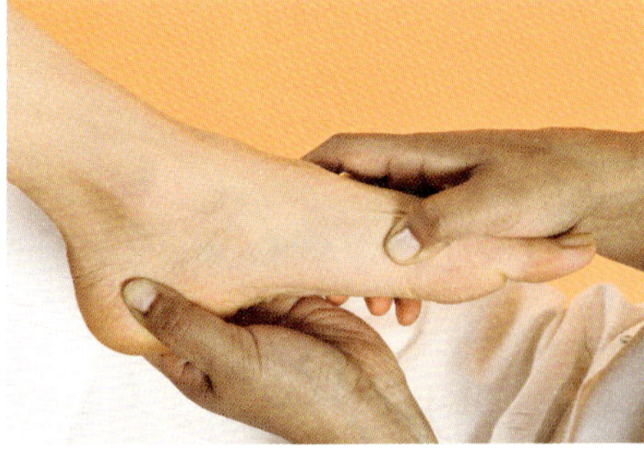

***3.*** *Activate the side of the foot, the area that corresponds to the upper back. With your other thumb, press on the heel to massage the coccyx. This allows you to open the energy flow in the vertebrae.*

***2.*** *Press on the point that corresponds to the spinal column. One finger placed on the upper part of the foot to work the cervical bones and the other on the lower part of the foot to work the back. This massage is especially good for tense muscles caused by straining activity.*

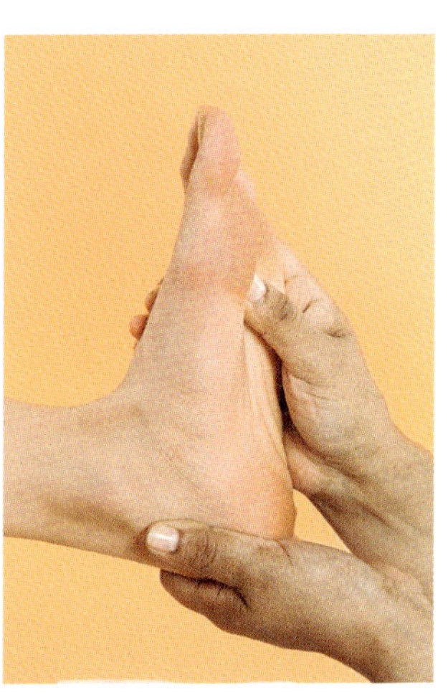

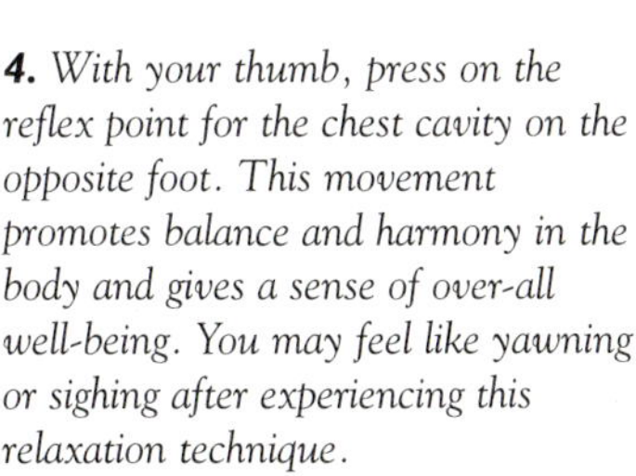

***4.*** *With your thumb, press on the reflex point for the chest cavity on the opposite foot. This movement promotes balance and harmony in the body and gives a sense of over-all well-being. You may feel like yawning or sighing after experiencing this relaxation technique.*

## PAY ATTENTION TO YOUR BODY

*Because tiredness can cause a number of symptoms, it is important to consider the messages the entire body sends to relieve the aches and ailments caused by exhaustion. Locate the reflex points in the feet that correspond to sore or tired parts of your body and apply pressure. The most effective and relaxing points tend to be the chest cavity, head, heart, shoulders and any other muscle or organ that is achy.*

# Color to make you feel better

Color therapy is a set of principles used to create harmonious color for healing. According to the principles of this therapy, color is energy. This form of energy medicine is based on the belief that the human body is composed of energy fields. This therapy stimulates the nerve centers and works on problems related to energy deficiencies which may cause physical and mental exhaustion.

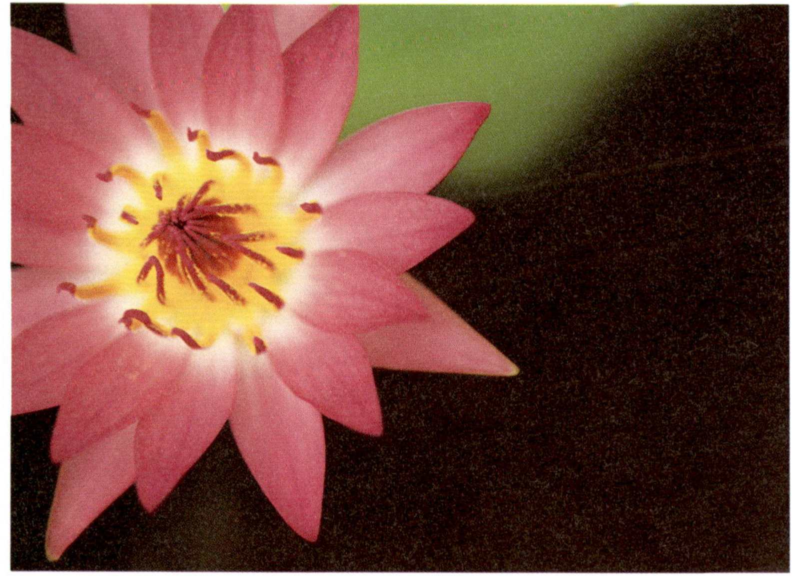

Well before science recognized the medical benefits of the ultraviolet and infrared wavelengths, natural healers used color therapy in treatment of patients. Greek philosopher Hippocrates said: *Human beings should harmonize the body and spirit.*
Today, natural medicine and color therapy are based on properly distributing energy.

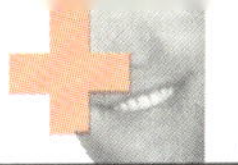

## COLOR AS TREATMENT

A typical color therapy session is done in a dark room, with colored optical slides, cromotherapy lamps or a simple slide projector. Colored light might be applied to parts of the recipient's body or to his entire body. The person recieving this therapy should be relaxed and focused on the color applied. The lights may be used constantly or rhythmically. The technique of solarized water is a simple and cheap way of applying color to the body. Water, when exposed to sunlight in a colored container for at least an hour becomes irradiated and takes on some of the vibrational energy of that particular color. Using this same method you can also prepare solarized sugar or oil.

### The power of colors

All colors, depending on their characteristics have curing powers, and each color is applied for varying ailments.

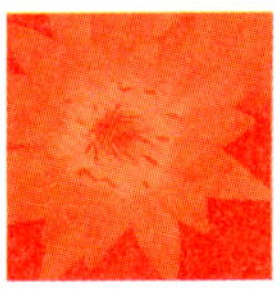

**Red.** Activates the circulatory system. Stimulates the process of learning and concentration; increases your will power and constancy.

• Ideal for fighting against weariness in the body, especially when you are experiencing tiredness in general. It is recommended to incorporate red into a room used for study for ideal concentration and creativity. It is also recommended if you need to study, write, read or do any intellectual task and feel tired.

**FOR EACH *CHAKRA*, A COLOR**

Oriental disciplines have for centuries considered *chakras* centers of energy. Each *chakra* corresponds to a certain color of lights applied to that point to balance the body's natural energy.

- *Chakra* on the crown of the head: **violet.**
- *Chakra* of the third eye, in the center of the forehead: **indigo.**
- *Chakra* of the throat: **turquoise, blue** and **sky blue.**
- *Chakra* of the heart: **green.**
- *Chakra* of the chest cavity: **yellow.**
- *Chakra* of the suprarenal glands: **red.**
- *Chakra* of the reproductive organs: **orange.**

**Orange.** Useful for nervous exhaustion. Lifts up the spirit and leaves a sense of euphoria.

• If you lead a sedentary life, incorporating this color into your surroundings can stimulate your willpower, lift you up and make you want to get up and move around.

**Yellow.** Relaxes the muscles and reduces excess worry when you are under pressure.

• Helps in situations when you are pessimistic or unsatisfied. Using yellow clothing during the day can lift up your energy and sleeping in a yellow room will help you to wake up in the morning.

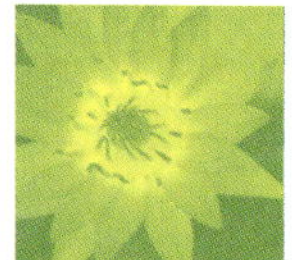

**Green.** Regenerates the body's cells, relaxes the muscles and relieves tired sight. Soothes tensions and aggressions and renews optimism.

• This pain relieving color can be used to calm aches and pains. This is an ideal color for a room you use for rest.

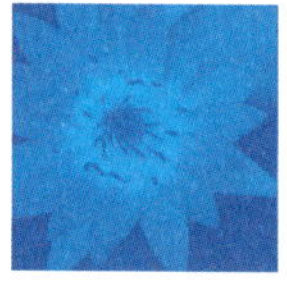

**Blue.** This color gives a sense of relaxation and restfulness. Helps to get over fears.

• A massage under blue light can help to relieve pain and gives immediate results. Helps you to recover from tiredness and makes other therapies like massages more effective.

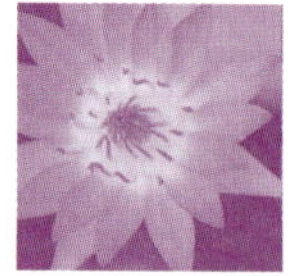

**Violet.** Detoxifies the body, supporting the expulsion of toxins and improving oxygen flow to the cells. Stimulates brain activity.

• Stimulates blood flow to the brain, activating intuition and inspiration. This color is the perfect color in the place where

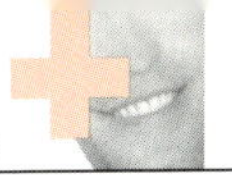

you must work hard and use brain power, because it reduces stress and tension.

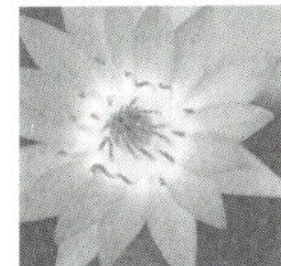

**White.** Fortifies the immune system. Produces a state of positive energy and good spirits.
Enlivens and empowers other color rays. It is the best color for inside your house to maintain a calm spirit and a constant energy.

## INCORPORATE COLOR IN YOUR LIFE

Knowing the properties of color you can use them in your daily life to activate your vital energy when you are tired. Using colors depends on your creativity and personal taste. Some alternatives for using colors include:

- Decorative paintwork on the walls of your home.
- Clothes and accessories.
- Filtered lamps that reflect different tones.
- Objects or adornments with stones or colored crystals.
- Choosing foods for their colors.

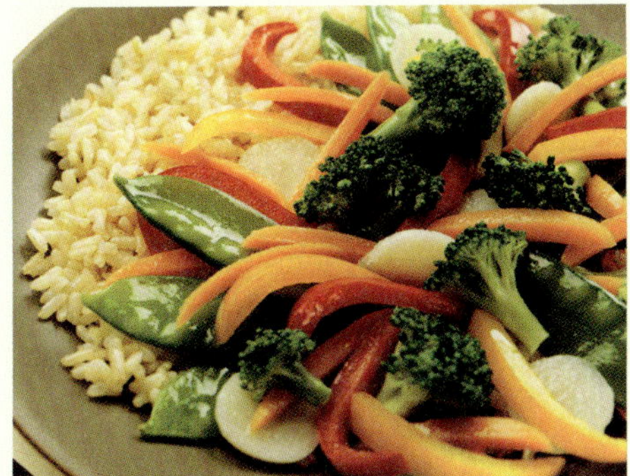

- Paintings of landscapes –or landscapes to visit– where certain colors predominate.

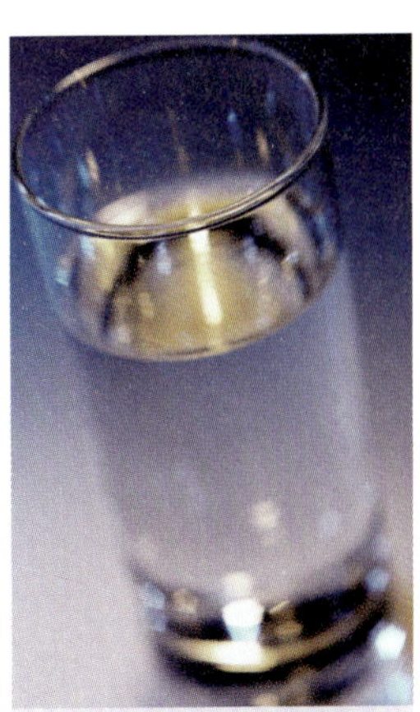

**RECIPE FOR CHARGED WATER**

**Place mineral water or spring water in a bottle of the color which you need, or improvise with a clear bottle covered with colored cellophane. Expose the water to sunlight from the morning until dusk and then store in a dark place. Water is used to treat different problems. It can be taken in a dose of 3 tablespoons a day, preferably before meals or during fasts. Children can take up to 2 spoonfuls a day.**

# Water, flowing with energy

Since ancient times water has been used as a natural medicine to cure the human body. Hydrotherapy is the use of water at different temperatures to revitalize, maintain, and restore health. There are a number of hydrotherapy techniques that use cold or hot water to stimulate the nervous system and to soothe pain.

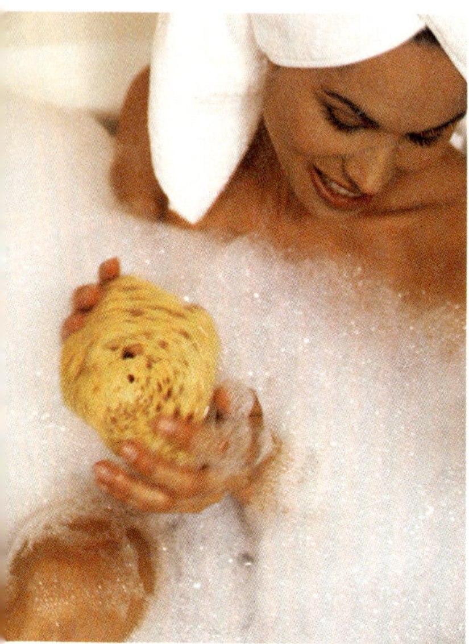

Water is considered by Chinese medicine to be one of the five basic elements that carry curative properties for the body and the soul. Ancient cultures in the East and West have used water for its curative properties: the bath has been used as a ritual to eliminate impurities in almost all religions.

## HYDROTHERAPY TO FIGHT FATIGUE

Taking a cold or hot water bath with essential oils or herbs provides incredible therapeutic effects. Other techniques include soaking, washing, rubbing and compresses.

**WARNING**

You should always consult your physician before starting any alternative treatment. If you suffer from high blood pressure, you should not use cold water.

### Bath

Depending on your energy level and physical state there are different water temperatures you can use.

- **Cold water.** Increases your sensitivity, shrinks your blood vessels, stimulates your blood pressure and tones the nervous system.
- **Warm or hot water.** Relaxes tense muscles and supports the immune system.

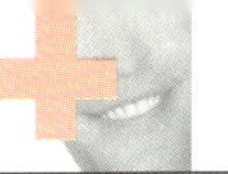

If you take a shower its best to:

- If it is cold, remain under the water for five minutes.
- If the water is hot or warm, stay in the shower for fifteen minutes.

If you are soaking in a bath, it's recommended:

- If you use warm water to restore your energy and improve circulation, stay in the water for five minutes and then exercise so that you warm up or rest in a warm bed.
- If you use warm water to relax and to relieve achy muscles, stay in the water for ten minutes.
- You can also add the bath salts or essential oils recommended for resting to the bath (see *Essential oils from A to Z*, on page 47).

**Warning.** It's advisable to avoid these types of baths if you suffer from low blood pressure.

**FOOT BATH**

**This is an ideal therapy to relieve tired feet and legs. You should fill a bucket with cold water, high enough so that you soak your legs. As with baths, you can add essential oils to the water to help you rest. Soak your feet and legs for a minute. Remove your legs from the water, dry off and cover your feet with cotton socks and rest for a while.**

## SPRAY SHOWERS

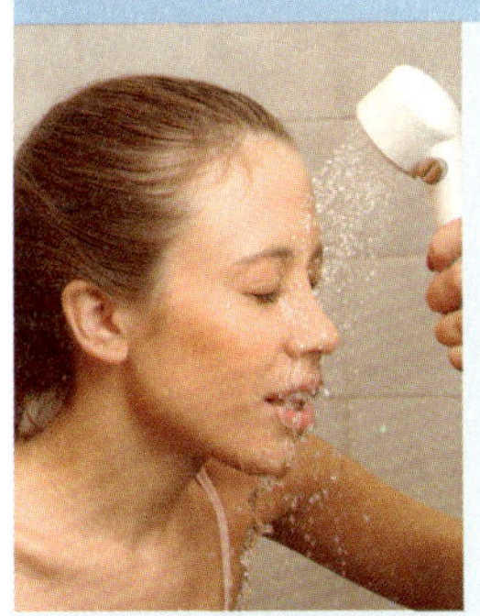

This is a type of massage using shower jets to apply pressure. It helps to tone the muscles, stimulate oxygen flow to the muscle tissues, increases the skin's resistance, stimulates circulation and, more than anything, helps to rejuvenate your body.

- **On the face.** This is a relaxing technique for the body and mind and it is perfect for treating headaches and migraines. Begin with the forehead, placing it under cold water and moving the water round in a clock-wise direction. Don't stop breathing, breathe through your mouth.

- **On the arms.** This is a shower technique that will give you an instant pick-me-up, because it activates circulation and stimulates deep breathing.

**1.** Begin by passing the cold waterjet on your right hand along the outter part of the right arm and move up until your shoulder, leaving it under the water for a few minutes.

**2.** Next, run the inner part of you arm under cold water, from your triceps to the palm of your hand. Repeat on the left side.

For cases of tiredness and lack of concentration, use this shower therapy on your arms, alternating between warm and cold water.

# Relieving aromas

Aromatherapy uses essential oils extracted from herbs and plants as a technique to care for the body. Essential oils can be used for their aromas and can be applied to soften the skin and penetrate the skin pores. This therapy restores the nervous system and leaves one in a highly relaxing state.

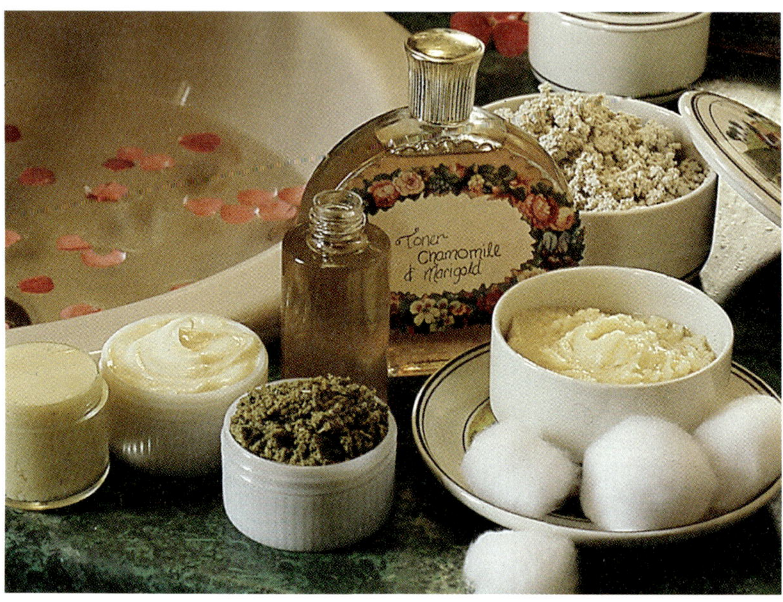


Essential oils can be used in order to balance physical, psychological and spiritual symptoms. Their aromas affect the sense of smell while smoothly penetrating through your skin and revitalizing your nervous system. Essential oils can be added to baths, salves and used in massages to relieve tiredness and other ailments. We have put together a list of *Essential oils from A to Z*, on page 47. Following the list are several recipes for home treatments against fatigue.

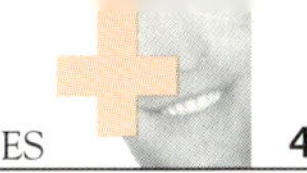

## ANGELICA TO CLEAR THE MIND

Wherever you study, read or meditate prepare an aromatherapy clay pot with 3-5 drops of angelica essential oil to improve your concentration. This oil can be even more potent when mixed with patchouli.

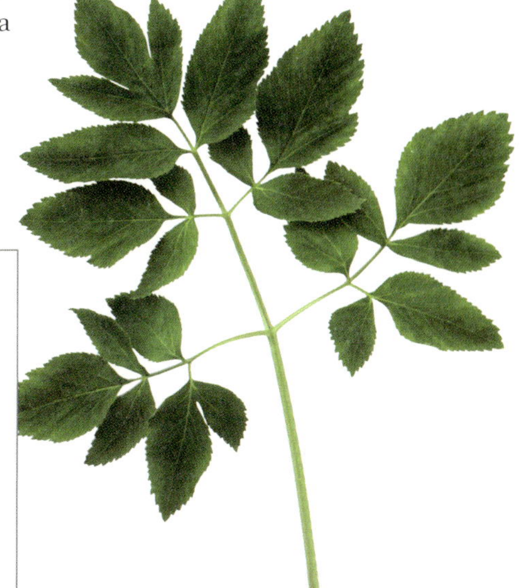

### INVIGORATING BATH

*Add 10 drops of angelica oil to a warm bath and soak away. This aroma gives a sense of confidence and balances the mind. It is recommended to use this therapy when you have to make an important decision.*

## JUNIPER

Sleepy bath: dilute 10 drops of this essential oil to a filled bath tub. After soaking you will feel calm and relief from tensions and tiredness.

### ANTI-DEPRESSIVE AROMATHERAPY

*Place an opened bottle of juniper oil close to your face and leave it there for a few minutes while you continue breathing normally to absorb the aroma. Next, place the bottle close to the solar plexus, continuing to breathe. Immediately you will feel energized and your mood will improve.*

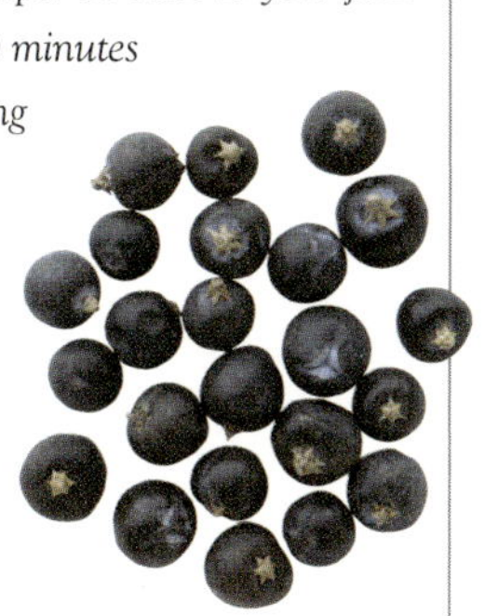

### RESTFUL BATHS

**Dilute 10 drops of essential oil of juniper to a bathtub. In addition, add 3 or 4 drops of essential oil of mandarin or camomile, to help you recover from sleepiness or mental exhaustion.**

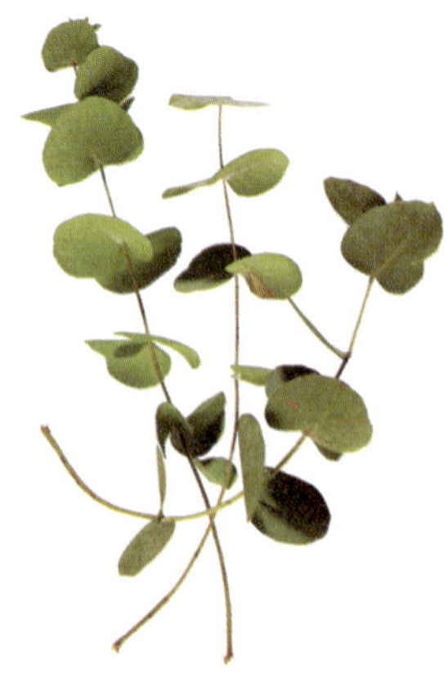

## EUCALYPTUS TO CLEAN YOUR BODY AND YOUR HOME

This essential oil can be used to relax or purify spaces where you've had arguments or experienced stress. Prepare a spray bottle with 10 drops of eucalyptus oil and 2 cups of spring water. Spray the room and your face with this aromatic water.

## GINGER CALMING MASSAGES

Essential oil of ginger is very effective to relieve tension when used in massages. This oil has very potent properties that stimulate the blood flow. It should always be diluted because it can irritate the skin. Its sedative effect can calm sore muscles caused by fatigue; to treat achy muscles massage a few drops directly onto the sore area.

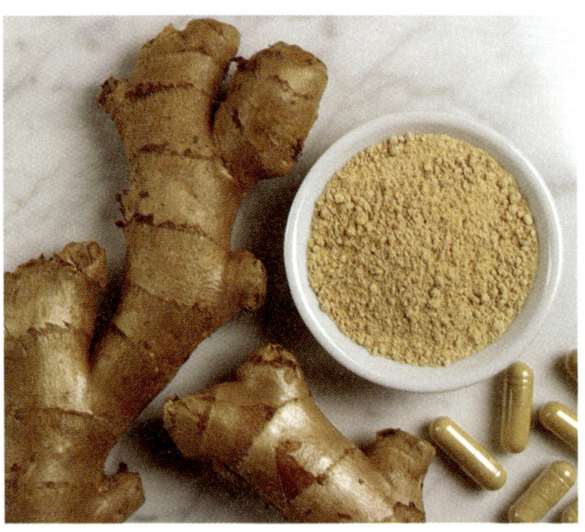

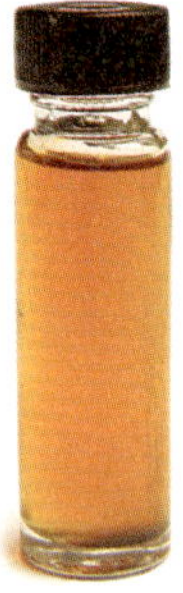

## LIMONCELLO OR LEMON HERB TO REST AT NIGHT

At night, dilute 4 drops of lemon oil in an aromatherapy clay pot, to recover from an exhausting day and to help relax and enjoy evening activities like reading.

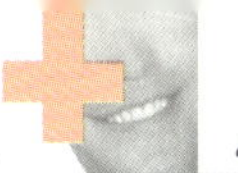

## LEMON TO IMPROVE STUDY

Dilute a few drops of lemon oil in a spray bottle with a small amount of water and spray the room where you are going to read or study. This aroma can improve your concentration.

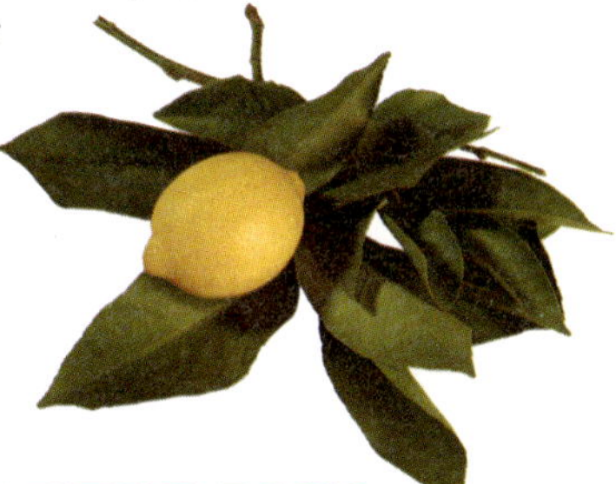

## ROMAN CAMOMILE RESTFUL BALM

Dilute a few drops of camomile with a bit of water and moisten linen cloths to use as compresses for sore or fatigued muscles.

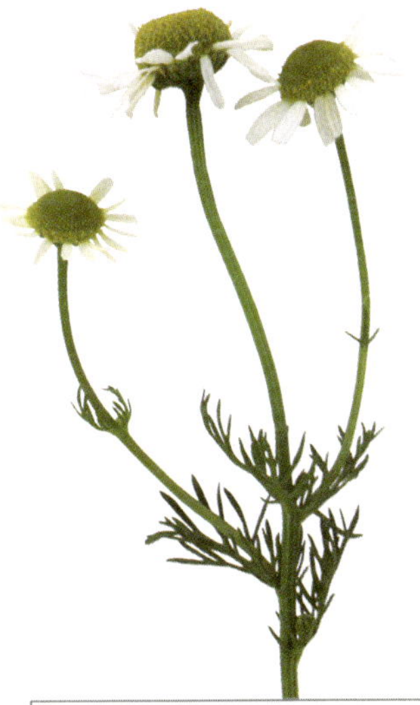

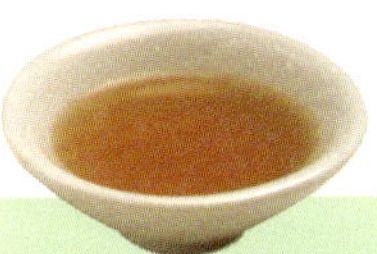

**RELAXING BATH**

**Add a few drops of camomile oil to a warm bath, soaking in this fragranced water will help you get away from your worries and rest.**

**FOR YOUR FEET**

**Apply pressure to reflexology points on your feet, using essential oil of camomile. This will relax and calm your spirit, helping to change your mood.**

### RELAXING MASSAGES

*Add a few drops of essential oil of camomile in a small bottle with sweet almond oil and use for back and abdominal massages. This therapy is great for when you are feeling oversensitive; this oil is ideal for fighting against insomnia and anxiety.*

## NIAULI PURIFING

This oil is useful if you work at home. It's advised to "purify" the energy that charges the room, which can interfere with rest. Dilute a few drops of niauli oil in a spray bottle with water and spray the room. This essence lifts up your spirits and energizes. Because it's a strong fragrance, you may want to mix a few drops of geranium oil, which stimulates positive thinking.

### ESSENCE BLENDS

**Formulas to pick you up**

Use a clay pot in a room you can relax in after a strenuous day at work. Here are two of the most efficient formulas:

- 3 drops of lemon, 3 drops of orange, 4 drops of bergamot.
- 3 drops of lavender, 4 drops of cedar, 3 drops of orange.

## PINE VAPORS TO FIGHT FATIGUE

Add 7 drops of pine essence to 2 cups of hot water. Put a towel over your head and tilt your head over the bowel and inhale for 15 minutes.

**Warning.** Before using this oil it's best to test your sensitivity, applying a small amount on your skin and leaving it for 15 minutes to make sure it doesn't irritate your skin or cause an allergic reaction.

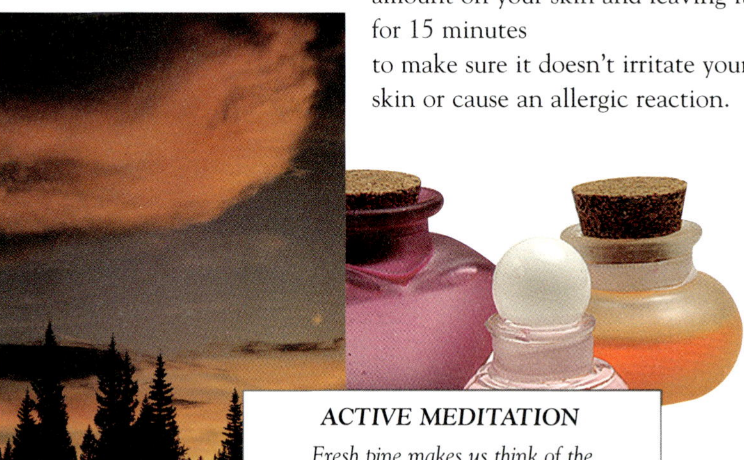

### ACTIVE MEDITATION

*Fresh pine makes us think of the mountains. Add a few drops to a clay pot for aromatherapy; sit or lie down in a comfortable position, close your eyes and visualize a forest. This essence evokes a sense of peace and erases daily exhaustion.*

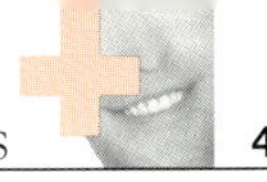

WARNING

*Aromatherapy clay pots shouldn't be used for more than two hours, because prolonged exposure to fragrance can cause headaches or neutralize the therapeutic effect of each essential oil.*

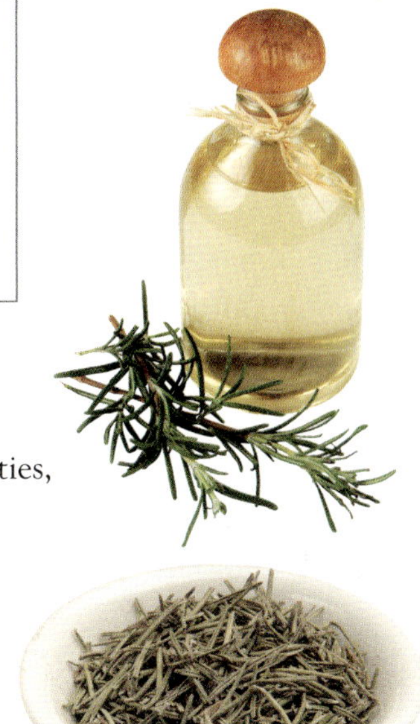

## ROSEMARY MOTIVATING BATH

This herb has gently euphoric properties, indicated in cases of psychological problems for those who feel disappointed or unable to achieve their objectives. Add a cup of rosemary infusion to a warm bath. You will feel energized and optimistic.

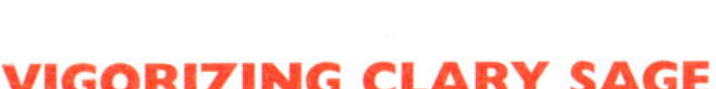

## VIGORIZING CLARY SAGE

Draw up a warm bath, add a few drops of clary sage essence and soak in the bath no longer than 15 minutes.
Clary sage produces a sense of euphoria and calms anxiety. Because this bath therapy can make it difficult to concentrate, you shouldn't drive afterward. It's best to use clary sage before going to bed, because it can induce sleep.

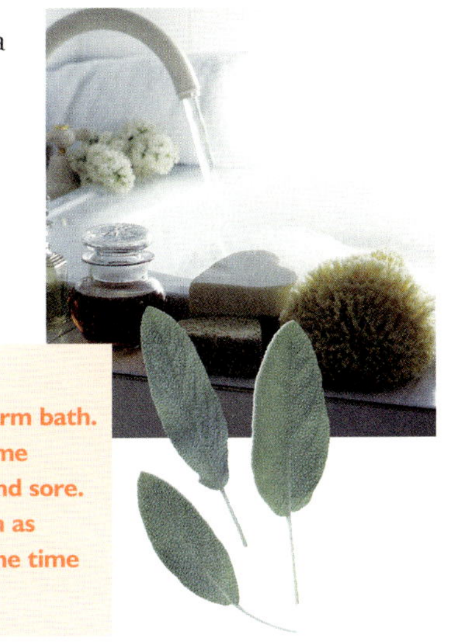

### REVITALIZING CLARY SAGE

**Add a few drops of sage essential oil to a warm bath. This oil can be used for cases of extreme exhaustion, when the body feels fatigued and sore. In Chinese medicine this herb is known as a *yin* tonic, because it calms and at the same time stimulates the nervous system.**

# Herbs and essentials to relax

Medicinal herbs can be taken as infusions or capsules to fight tiredness. While essential oils, also made from herbs can be used in aromatherapy. In the following pages, we have developed a guide of the most efficient plants that work as remedies for tiredness and a list of essential oils from A to Z, that when used externally can help fight fatigue.

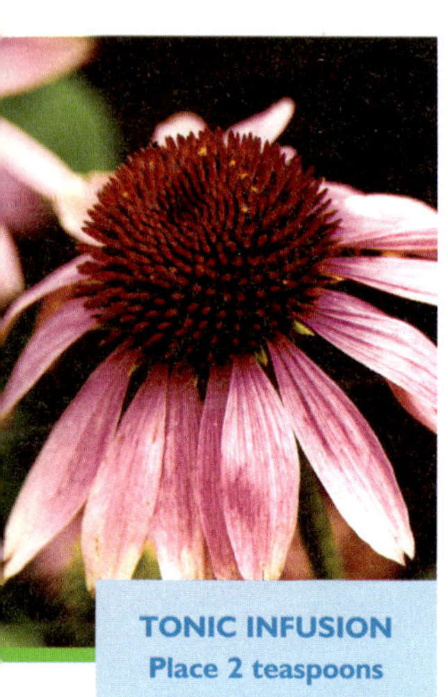

**TONIC INFUSION**
Place 2 teaspoons of dried echinacea in 1 cup with boiling water. Let steep for 5 minutes, drain and drink.

## Echinacea

*(Echinacea purpurea and Echinacea angustifolia)*

- **Parts used.** The root and flowers are used. Powdered echinacea and tincture are made from the plant's roots. Relatively recently, the flowers began to be used to make capsules.
- Echinacea is a wild flower native to North America. Native Americans used the plant for a variety of conditions, including high fevers and venomous bites.
- This is one of the most widely used natural remedies in the West, because of its antiviral and antibacterial properties. It supports and stimulates the body's immune system.
- It is not known what causes echinacea's curative actions, but it can be used in cases of fatigue for its stimulating-tonic properties.

## Ginkgo Biloba

*(Ginkgo biloba)*

**NOTE**
You should always consult your physician before starting any herbal treatment.

- **Parts used.** The seeds and leaves are used in homemade infusions, which haven't been proven effective. However, it has been demonstrated that ginkgo extracts and capsules made from the plant's leaves are very effective.

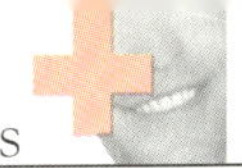

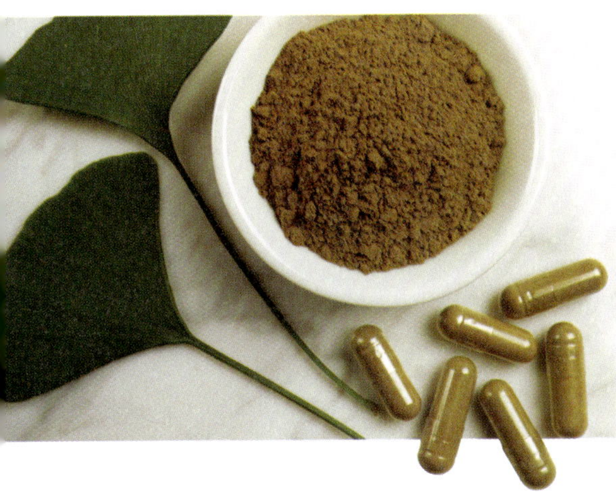

You can find them in health food stores.

- The ginkgo tree species is native to China. During the Middle Ages, it was believed by Europeans that this tree came from the Garden of Eden.
- It is a powerful tonic for the mind. Ginkgo extract activates the metabolism of the brain, improving blood and oxygen circulation.
- Its active properties improve memory, lack of concentration, depression and other ailments related to fatigue.
- **Warning.** Although this plant doesn't have serious side effects, the seeds can be toxic. It's not recommended for children or the elderly to take this remedy. You shouldn't use the seeds, because their extract can be irritating.

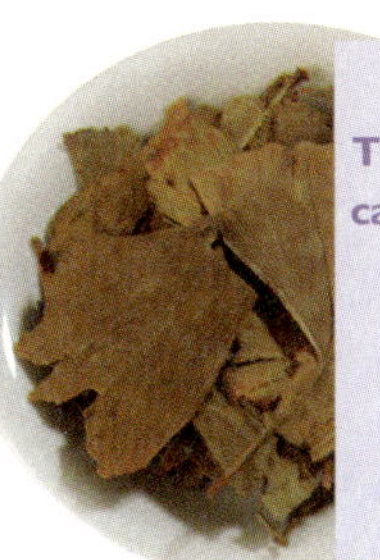

**RINGING IN YOUR EARS**

**This persistent and bothersome symptom can be caused by insufficient circulation in the brain. This ailment can cause headaches, exhaustion and fatigue. Take 80 to 120 mg of ginkgo extract capsules a day, always under medical supervision.**

## ESSENTIAL OILS FROM A TO Z

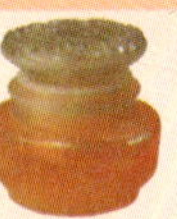

### ANGELICA

Stimulates the nervous system, relieves fatigue and improves concentration. Use in baths, vapors, massages and compresses. It blends well with clary sage and lemon.

**Safety.** Excessive use can have a narcotic effect and decrease blood circulation. Can be toxic in high doses. It increases your photo-sensibility, making it important to avoid direct sunlight after using.

### CLARY SAGE

This potent sedative can be used in vapors.

It releases tensions that prevent the free flow of energy. It also calms the nerves and clears the mind. As it helps to awaken contemplation, it is good for meditation.

**Safety.** It should be used in low doses, because it can be soporific.

**WARNING**

Essential oils are for external use **only**, they should **never** be ingested. Keep stored away from children and keep away from your eyes.

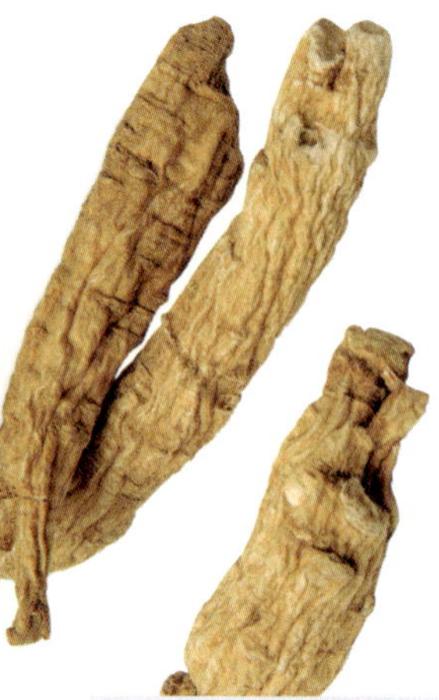

**FOR MORE ENERGY**
It's recommended to take 1-2 tablets of Siberian ginseng once a day, always under medical supervision.

**ENERGETIC TONIC**
For a lasting effect, prepare a decoction with guarana seed. Prepare by adding 2 teaspoons of crushed guarana seeds to 1 cup of boiling water and let steep for 5 minutes. Drain and drink 2 or 3 cups a day.

## Siberian ginseng
*(Eleutheroccoccus senticosus)*

• **Parts used.** The roots. Fresh or dried Siberian ginseng root is not available on the market, you can only buy it in capsule form, made from a base of the root.

• Stimulating effects that increase physical and mental stamina, especially for cases of extreme exhaustion.

• There are three varieties of this plant, but when it is used in Chinese medicine it is used in particular for cases of energy deficiency, or lack of vital energy in the heart. It also has physical therapeutic effects, calming heart palpitations, supporting the immune system and assisting the body in tolerating aggressions.

• **Warning.** Do not take ginseng continuously for more than four weeks. It can cause insomnia and high blood pressure. It's best to avoid coffee or caffeinated tea while using ginseng. You should not take this remedy if you are healthy, only take it if you have signs of tiredness or physical fatigue. This remedy is not recommended for pregnant women or for children under 12 years old.

## Guarana
*(Paulina cupana)*

• **Parts used.** The seeds, covered in a shell are toasted and ground to make a brown powder. The roots are also used.

• This plant native to the Amazon area, produces a seed rich in caffeine and other stimulating substances. The indigenous people of the Amazon rain forest use crushed guarana seed as a beverage and a medicine.

• Stimulates the central nervous system and promotes the release of adrenaline. Keeps your

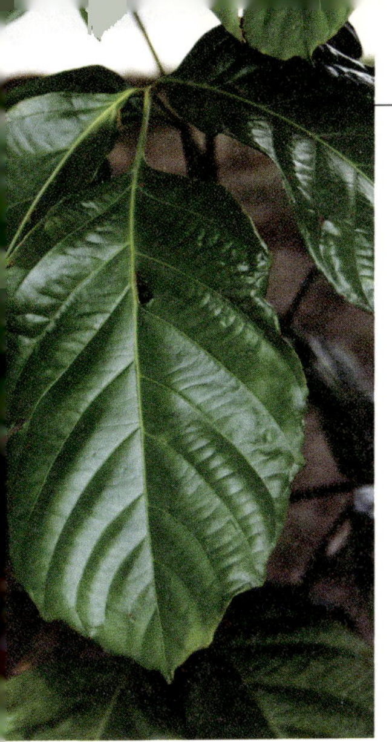

arteries clear, elastic, supporting good blood circulation in the body.

• Thanks to its caffeine content, it prolongs stamina and increases the body's capacity to use physical strength.

• It promotes the use of glucose in the muscles, benefiting the muscular tissue, increasing the muscle's stamina against fatigue. Used as a tonic and general stimulant, it fights against physical exhaustion, fatigue or low energy.

• Can be used in tablets (made with the dried extract) or in a powder to mix with juices and other liquids.

• It shouldn't be used with other stimulants (ginseng, coffee, maté, etc) or with tranquilizers.

• **Warning.** Avoid guarana if you suffer from caffeine intolerance, high blood pressure, serious cardiovascular disorders, ulcer and insomia. It shouldn't be taken during pregnancy and lactation. Avoid giving children guarana.

## A REMEDY FROM THE AMAZON

In the Amazon forest guarana is traditionally prepared by toasting the seeds to avoid fermentation. Natives use a traditional method of preparation by drying and roasting the seeds and mixing them with water to make a paste. The mixture is cooked over fire. This is called "guarana paste", which the indigenous people drink by placing it in a cup of hot water throughout the day as an energetic tonic.

## ESSENTIAL OILS FROM A TO Z

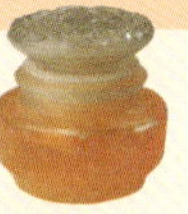

### EUCALYPTUS

Its aroma stimulates and clears the mind; strengthens the nervous system and immune function, increasing your body's defenses when you are tired or fighting an illness. It purifies the air and body. This potent aroma can be used in sprays, baths, compresses or massages; when using on the skin eucalyptus should be diluted.

**Safety.** Can irritate the skin. Shouldn't be used if you suffer from high blood pressure.

### GINGER

Intense stimulant that at the same time comforts and brings on a sense of euphoria, which can help to relieve states of extreme tiredness. This nervous tonic calms your emotions and improves your memory. It also has revitalizing effects, especially when used with other oils like ylang ylang, lavender and angelica. It can be added to baths, vapors, massages and compresses.

**Safety.** If you have sensitive skin, it is advised to use this oil diluted.

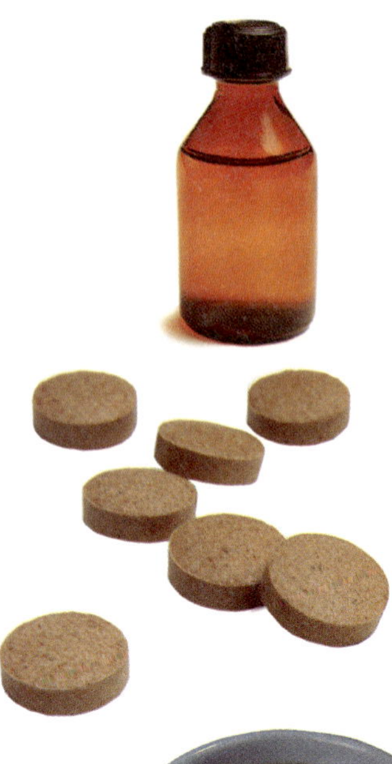

## Huang qi

*(Astragalus membranaceus)*

• **Parts used.** The roots are extracted from the plant when it is 4 to 7 years old; the roots are cultivated in the spring. It is used to prepare infusions, make capsules or tinctures, which can be found in most natural food stores.

• *Huan qi* in extracts strengthens the body's inmune system and increases the production of antibodies to fight off external cell destruction and tumor cells.

• *Chi* or essential energy tones the body. It is also called the factor of resistance because in Chinese medicine it is prescribed for cases of fatigue or weakness.

• There are three ways to take *huang qi*: decoction of fresh or dried root; in capsules or tablets made from dried extract of the plant; in tincture (made with alcohol maceration).

• **Warning.** Do not take with other stimulants, like gingseng, coffee, tea or maté.

**Recommended dose:**

• Take 3 to 5 teaspoons of fresh root per day in a decoction.

• Supplements usually contain 500 mg of *huang qi*. Take 2 or 3 capsules per day.

• Tincture, take 1 teaspoon 3 times a day.

### FIGHTING TIREDNESS

Prepare a decoction of the bark, placing 1 tablespoon of the bark in 2 cups of cold water and let boil 5 to 15 minutes. Filter and drink throughout the day.

## Pink trumpet tree

*(Tabebuia avellanedae)*

• **Parts used.** The internal bark that is

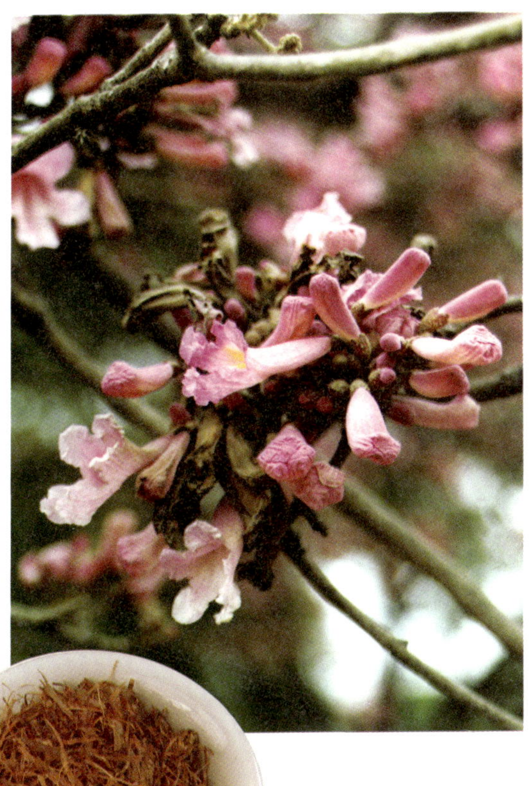

collected from wild trees, to prepare in decoctions, medicinal tinctures and salves.

- This tree, native to South America, is valued for its hard wood and its curative properties for treating complex ailments like post-viral fatigue, recuperating from an illness, loss of energy and fighting cancer with coadjutant treatments.
- Many of its components stop the growth of tumors, by impeding their metabolism of oxygen.
- Because of its properties it is used to restore a body tired out by fatigue.

## ESSENTIAL OILS FROM A TO Z

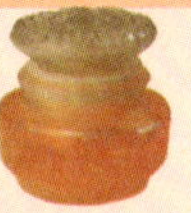

### JUNIPER

Its stimulant properties clear and tone the mind. Especially good if you are under a lot of pressure or with a lot of responsibilities, if you feel tired or if you feel anxious or antsy. Excellent antidepressant, this oil develops the spirit's harmony; its fresh aroma lifts up your spirits and improves your self-esteem. It blends well with geranium, lavender and vetiver.

**Safety.** Shouldn't be used during pregnancy, because excessive use can bring on birth. High doses and concentrates can irritate the skin.

### LEMON

Used to treat psychological symptoms of tiredness because it clears and refreshes the mind, increasing concentration, improving energy and emotional well-being. Blend with incense, ylang ylang or camomile.

**Safety.** This essence can irritate the skin if it isn't diluted. Because of its photo-toxic effects it's best to avoid exposure to sunlight after using it.

## Kola nut

*(Cola acuminata)*

• **Parts used.** The seeds are used to make powder or tincture. The powder or seeds are used in infusion or tincture form diluted with water.

• This majestic tree is native to Africa where it has been used as a medicinal remedy and aphrodisiac.

• General stimulant that tones the nervous system and heart. It also helps to recover energy.

• Used for cases of psychological and physical fatigue and for nervous depression.

• **Warning.** Although this is a stimulant for the nervous system, in high doses it can have a depressing effect; it can produce over-excitement followed by depression.

**Recommended doses:**

• Infusion of powder made from seeds. Up to 1/2 teaspoon per cup.

• Seed infusion. Use one teaspoon per cup of tea. Drink 2 cups a day before meals.

• In tincture form. Drink up to 30 drops diluted in a glass of water, 3-4 times a day.

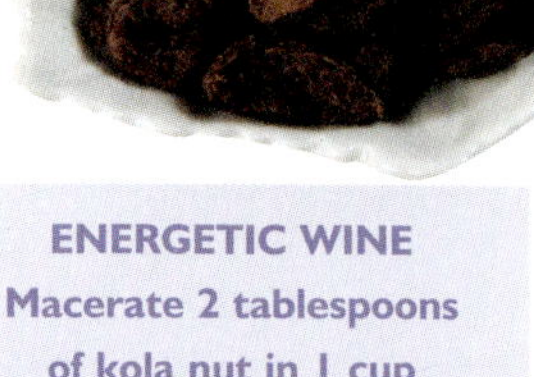

**ENERGETIC WINE**

Macerate 2 tablespoons of kola nut in 1 cup of high grade alcohol (in general 30 grades). After mixing add 3 cups of wine spirits and allow to age for 3 months. Filter and drink 3 small cups a day as a general tonic.

## Rosemary

*(Rosmarinus officinalis)*

• **Parts used.** The leaves, fresh or dried are used in infusions. They are also used to make essential oils and medicinal tinctures.

• Native to the Mediterranean, it was used in ancient culture to improve and strengthen the memory.

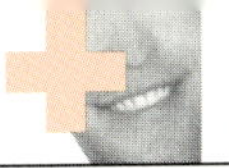

• Used for cases of tiredness, stress and slight depression.
• Its aroma and flavor is penetrating and is used in cooking. It is said that rosemary "lifts up the spirit."
• Stimulates blood pressure, especially in the head, improving concentration. It also helps to relieve headaches, improves memory and restores and invigorates the body after a long tiring day.

## FOR EXHAUSTION

• **Infusion for headache.** Take every 3 hours, 2 tablespoons of rosemary infusion prepared with dried leaves.

• **Revitalizing tincture.** Drink I teaspoon of tincture diluted in water, 2 times per day. It is an excellent tonic for the body.

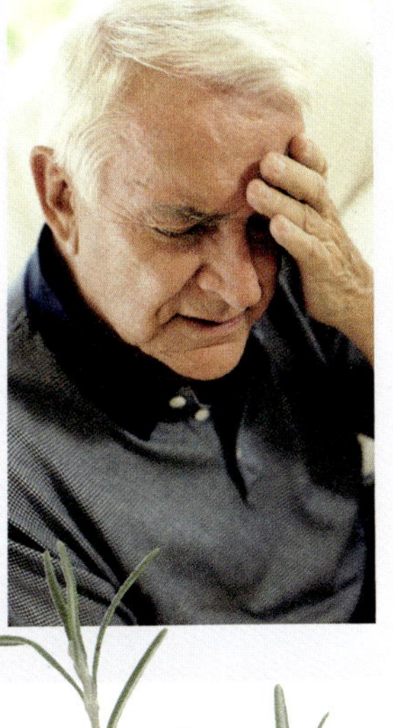

## ESSENTIAL OILS FROM A TO Z

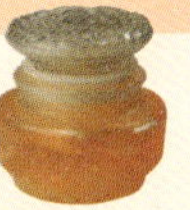

### LIMONCELLO OR LEMON HERB

Strengthens the body, and acts as an excellent muscular stimulant. This herb also helps to relieve the nervous exhaustion produced by tiredness. It also is good for headaches and exhaustion brought on by change of routines. Its aroma acts as a natural antidepressant. It can be blended with ginger and jasmine for a potent remedy. **Safety.** If you use in baths and massages, it's important to use small doses because it can be irritating.

### NIAULI

Physical and mental stimulant. Its tonic effects improve concentration and clear thinking. It's one of the most beneficial essential oils and it doesn't present side effects. It doesn't irritate the skin, always use high quality oil. **Safety.** Because of its stimulant characteristics, it's best to use it in the afternoon, combined with other sedative oils, such as lavender and fennel so that it doesn't cause insomnia.

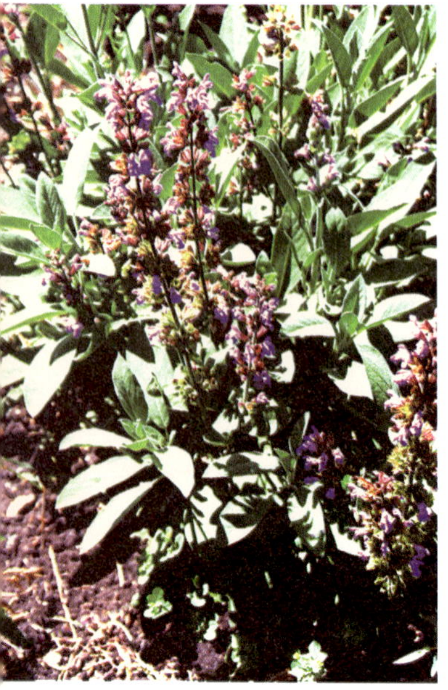

## Sage

*(Salvia officinalis)*

• **Parts used.** The leaves, fresh or dried are used to make infusions, essential oils and medicinal tinctures.

• It is known as a plant used in cooking. In Mediterranean cuisine, the plant's native region, sage is a common herb. Its name is a key to its curative properties: it comes from the Latin word *salvare*, which means "to save."

• Its components act as a gentle stimulating tonic for the central nervous system, for which reason it gives relief for everyday tiredness.

• In Chinese medicine it is considered to be a yin tonic, which calms and at the same time stimulates the nervous system.

• **Warning.** Do not drink this remedy during pregnancy and breastfeeding, because it is a strong hormonal stimulant and one of its components, tuyona, disrupts the production of breast milk.

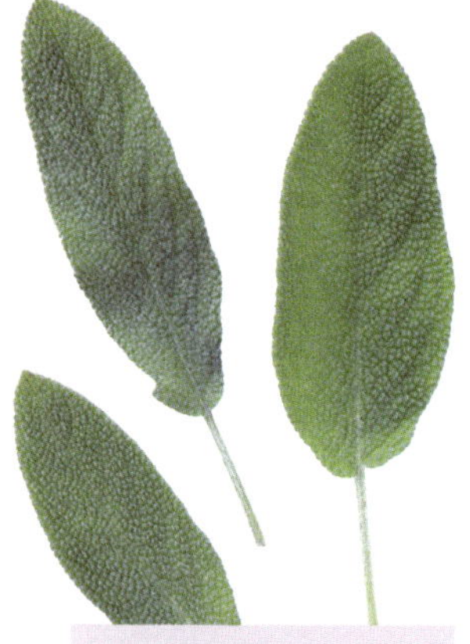

**FOR EVERYDAY EXHAUSTION**

Prepare an infusion with 1 tablespoon of sage flowers and leaves, add hot water to 1 cup, let sit for 5 minutes and strain. Drink 3 cups a day.

## Yerba maté

*(Ilex paraguaiensis)*

• **Parts used.** The leaves, which contain active components. It is cultivated by cutting the branches, which doesn't harm the tree.

• This plant species is native to the bordering regions of Argentina, Brazil and Paraguay. The indigenous people of this region, the Guarani, chewed on maté leaves during the day and would drink this herb as a comforting elixir that gives strength and energy.

• *Yerba maté* is a stimulant to fight mental and physical fatigue. It supports intellectual work.

*Yerba maté* contains vitamin C, complex B vitamins and minerals such as calcium, potassium and magnesium.

• It doesn't present any side effects except in cases of nervousness and insomnia.

**HOW TO DRINK YERBA MATÉ**

**This beverage can be used in two infusion forms:**

- **As a tea, by boiling water with 2 teaspoons of *yerba maté* (per cup) and draining before drinking.**
- **The most traditional way to drink *yerba maté* is in a small cup or gourd called *maté* through a *bombilla* (metal filter straw).**

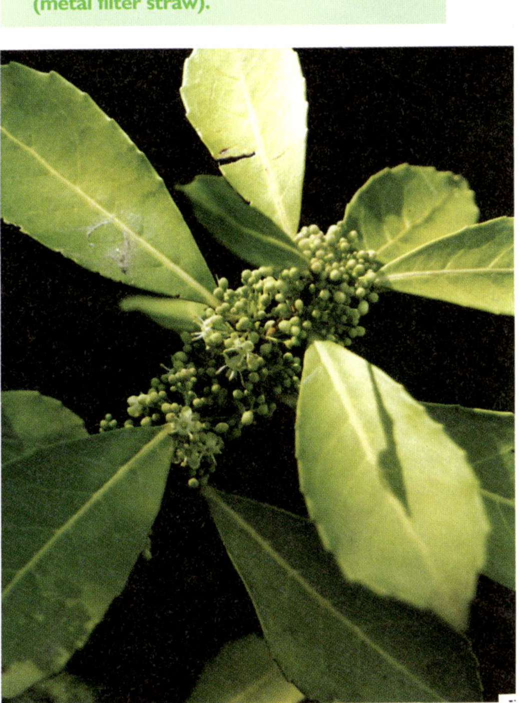

## ESSENTIAL OILS FROM A TO Z

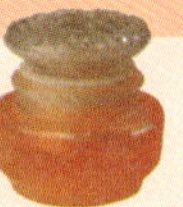

### PINE

Its balsamic properties restore and invigorate the mind. It is used for cases of low self-esteem and other psychological symptoms caused by fatigue.

**Safety.** This oil can cause allergic reactions for some people and bronchial spasms in children. When used in excess this oil can cause hypertension.

### ROMAN CAMOMILE

Powerful sedative for muscular pains caused by extreme tiredness. Its curative effects are not only physical but also psychological, because they are used for emotional problems caused by fatigue and stress. Can be combined with angelica and jasmine to make it more potent and to enrich a soft aromatic blend.

**Safety.** It shouldn't be used during the first four months of pregnancy.

# Foods to fight fatigue

Tiredness is one of the symptoms which indicates an imbalance of energy which is the product of various factors. Excessive activity, lack of rest, poor physical condition and daily pressures can cause tiredness, but an unbalanced diet can be a key element in not being able to recuperate.

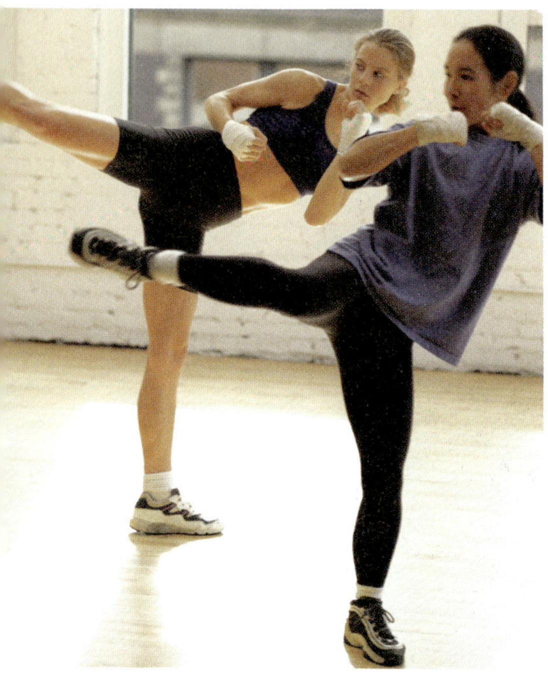

Our bodies act as motors and if we lack fuel (a lack of necessary nutrients) we feel tired and can end up getting fatigued or ill. Planning a balanced, nutrient diet rich in carbohydrates, proteins, minerals and vitamins is vital in fighting against extreme exhaustion. Iron rich foods like meat should be staples in your diet. You should also include a sufficient amount of vitamin C, found in fruits and vegetables, which can help to absorb iron and magnesium. A deficiency of magnesium can cause muscular weakness. At the same time it's advised to cut down on caffeine, which is a stimulating substance. Also, it is fundamental to drink enough liquids, at least 6 to 8 glasses of water per day. Calculate 3 to 5 glasses more for each hour of intense physical exercise, because dehydration can cause extreme fatigue.

## WHAT YOU CAN'T LACK

Because of their vital functions in providing energy, iron and zinc are the minerals for a diet to fight tiredness.

### Zinc

Essential for any age to maintain health, because it helps to support the break down of proteins, carbohydrates, fats and nucleic acids. It also helps to recharge energy after surgery and in cases of fever, states that tend to bring on cases of severe tiredness and chronic fatigue syndrome. A low level of zinc can aggravate illnesses, cause sleeping disorders, stunted growth, depression and loss of appetite. Found in **honey**, **fresh oysters**, **ginger**, **dried fruits**, **red meats** and **corn kernels**.

### Iron

Essential mineral for the formation of hemoglobin, that transports oxygen around the body, strengthens the immune system and prevents certain types of anaemia that can cause tiredness. In addition, this mineral intervenes in the production of energy enzymes. It increases the bones' resistance and helps to develop the intellectual capacity. Present in **honey**, **liver**, **brewers' yeast**, **grains**, **dried fruits**, **sardines**, **spinach**, **eggs** and **cauliflower**.

**NOTE**
**You should always consult your doctor before changing your diet.**

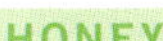

**HONEY**

Honey is a natural sugar, which is different from refined sugar, it provides calories rich in minerals, especially iron and zinc. It also contains vitamins in the complex B group, vitamin C, sodium, calcium, phosphorus, and magnesium. It helps to balance the body, acts as an energizing tonic and at the same time relaxes the nervous and circulatory system. Used for moments of mental and physical exhaustion. The key to honey is in its simple (mono sucrose) sugars, a powerful source of energy that the blood absorbs in its original form.

**DOSE AGAINST TIREDNESS**
**For cases of occasional fatigue and when recuperating from a prolonged illness it is recommended to take at least 4 teaspoons of honey a day, until you feel better. For slight cases of tiredness, take 1 teaspoon in the morning and another at night.**

## CARING FOR CHILDREN

- Children under one year old shouldn't ingest honey, because their intestinal flora is not stable. It can also increase the risk of allergies.
- For older children it is highly recommended, because it improves appetite and stimulates blood production and vigor. It also improves concentration.

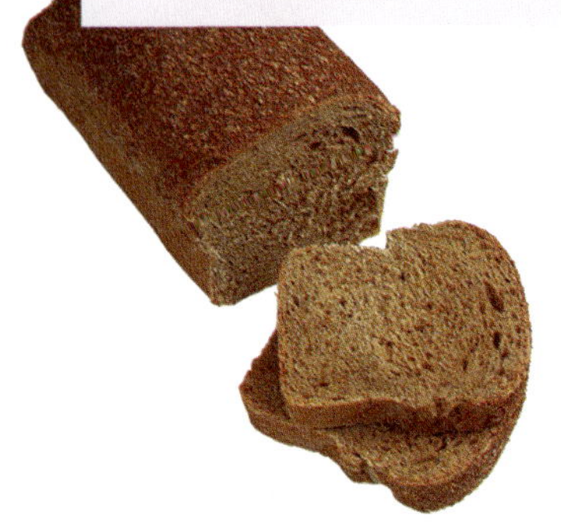

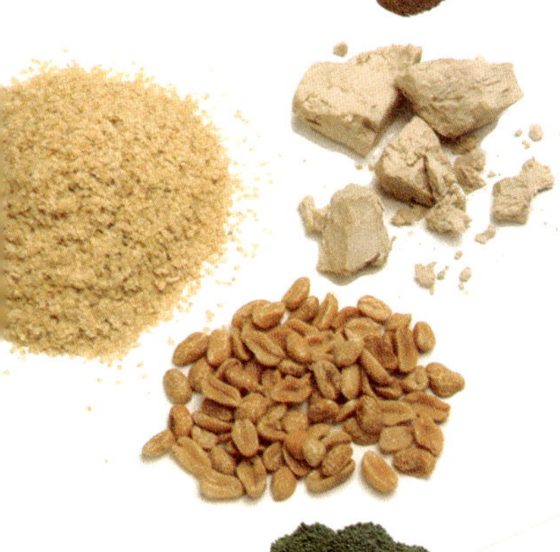

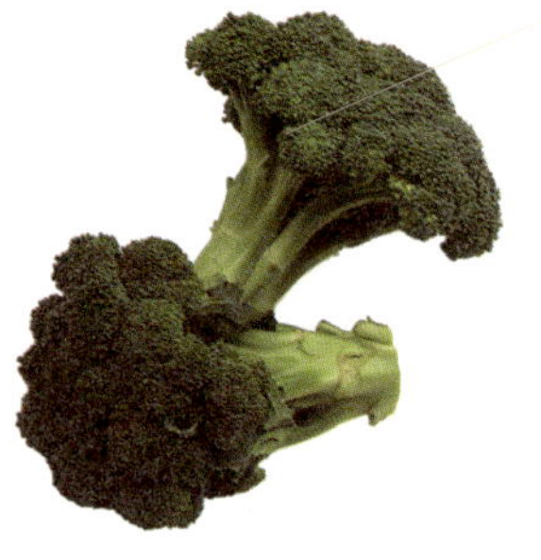

# VITAMINS AND MINERALS

## The vitamin B group

This vitamin group helps the functioning of the nervous system and the maintenance of mental health and metabolic energy. These vitamins are irreplaceable when recovering from exhaustion or fatigue.

■ $B_1$ Water-soluble nutrient that the body does not produce and needs to be incorporated into the diet. Helps to metabolize carbohydrates and improves digestion. Essential for energy, relieving states of tiredness and improving memory. Found in **sunflower seeds**, **beans**, **wholewheat breads**, **artichokes**, **celery**, **garlic** and other **vegetables**.

■ $B_2$ Helps to break down carbohydrates, proteins and fats, converting them into energy, this energy can be lost during periods of excessive tiredness. It also helps to protect the body against anaemia, migraines and cramping. It is found in **liver**, **almonds**, **dairy products** and **broccoli**.

■ $B_3$ The aminoacid tryptophan can be converted inside the human body to vitamin $B_3$, and is fundamental to produce energy. It contains enzymes that breakdown carbohydrates. It also regulates sugar in the blood, activates circulation, stimulates the nervous system and acts as an antioxidant.

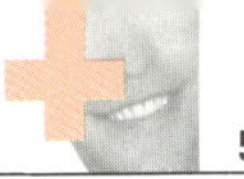

### *SESAME AGAINST FATIGUE*

*The body needs iron to produce the pigment that transports oxygen. Iron is found in the body's red blood cells and is fundamental for the formation of hemoglobin, a protein that transports oxygen. It supports the breathing of the body's cells. Vegetarians who don't consume animal products, rich in iron, can substitute sesame seeds, a source rich in iron and also containing calcium, zinc, foliate and complex B vitamins and vitamin E. You can toast sesame seeds in a pan and add them to meat and fish. This recipe is great for sprinkling over soups, stews and salads.*

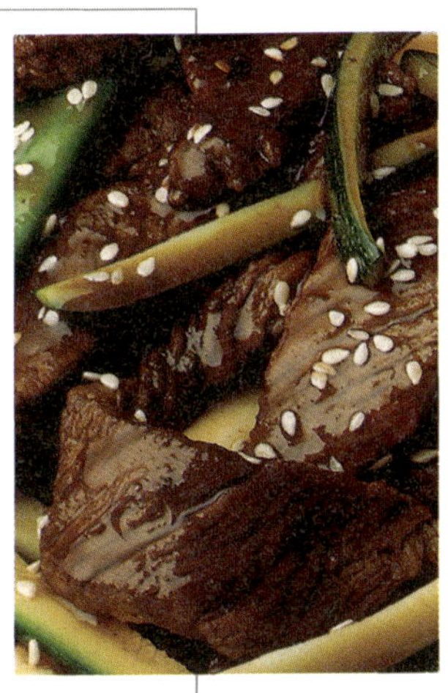

As with other B-complex vitamins it can be found in **wholegrain cereals**, **fish**, **eggs**, **dates**, **peanuts**, **milk** and **coffee**.

■ $B_4$ Acts in the functioning of supra-renal gland, which is activated when you are exhausted or under stress. It helps the body break down carbohydrates and proteins. It is helpful in cases of stress and exhaustion. Good sources of $B_5$ are **dairy products**, **eggs**, **peanuts**, **walnuts**, **avocado** and **lentils**.

■ $B_6$ It is an important vitamin for the immune system. It supports the metabolism, helps to balance hormones and breaks down fats and carbohydrates. It helps to prevent extreme tiredness and muscular cramps. It is found in **sunflower seeds**, **dried fruits**, **bananas**, **chicken** and **coffee**.

■ $B_{12}$ It's important for avoiding cases of fatigue and for maintaining the health of the nervous system, improving concentration and memory. It helps to prevent anaemia and to

**MEAT: IRON + VITAMIN B**

**Red meat is essential for iron and vitamin $B_{12}$, which is essential for the formation and maintenance of the nervous system, and helps increase your resistance to fatigue. Other meats, including fish and poultry, and eggs give similar benefits. They are rich in proteins, stimulate the brain and improve the mind's function.**

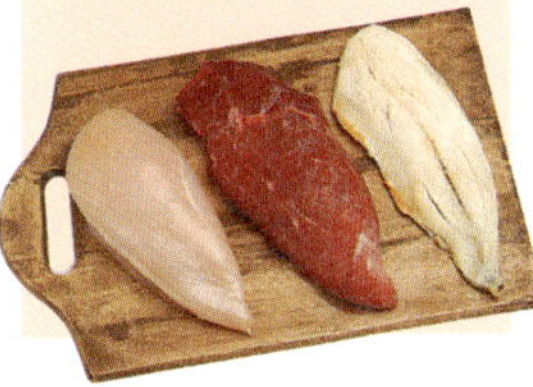

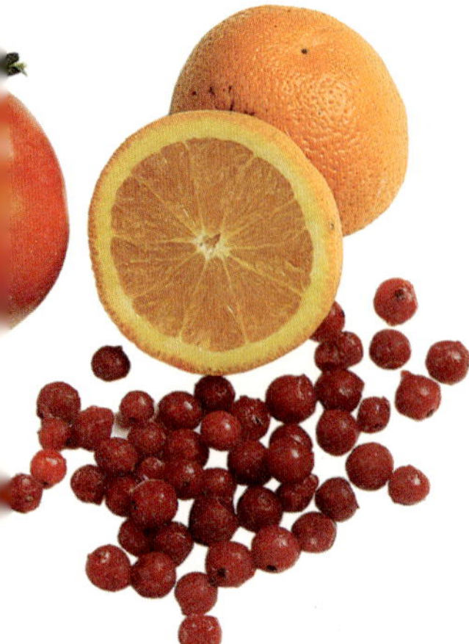

keep the body's health balanced. Found in **meat-derived** foods and some vegetables: **liver, oysters, salmon, eggs, cheese, fortified cereals** and **brewers' yeast.**

## Vitamin C

Prevents anaemia (because it helps to absorb iron), gastroduodenal ulcers and immune deficiencies. It is an anti-oxidant increasing the production of collagen, which helps to prevent premature aging. An anti-histamine, it is used for cases of allergies. **Warning.** Excess vitamin C supplements can provoke diarrhea. Found in **fruits** and **vegetables** like **apricots, lemon, broccoli, green** and **red peppers, potatoes, currants** and **guavas.**

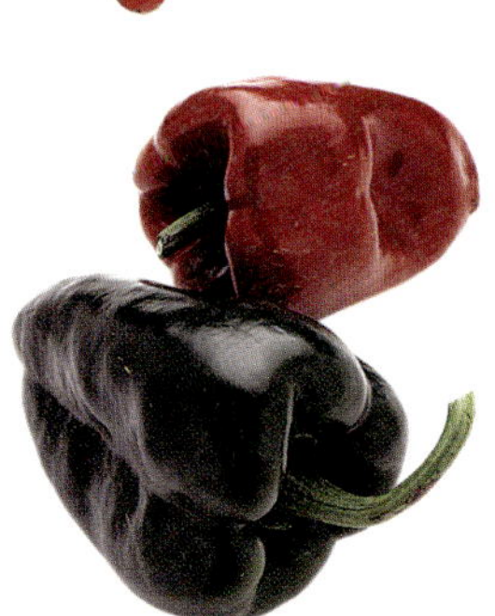

## Calcium

Promotes well-being, and excites the nerves and muscles. It also helps to relieve anxiety, regulate sleep and heart rhythm. Found in: **milk, cheese, yogurt, cider vinegar, sardines, leafy greens** and **sesame seeds.**

### LEMON

A citrus fruit, which is not eaten whole, but used in cooking and for medicinal and aesthetic remedies. Contains energizing components that activate the body's flow of fluids, which is good for cases of tiredness. Contains vitamin C, $B_1$ and $B_2$ and minerals such as potassium, calcium, magnesium and phosphorus.

**REMEDY FOR TIREDNESS**

**Juice 1 lemon, take out the seeds and add sugar and water. Drink to fight extreme fatigue, to give you an instant pick-me-up.**

**Safety. Those who suffer from gastritis or gastric acid should use lemon in moderation.**

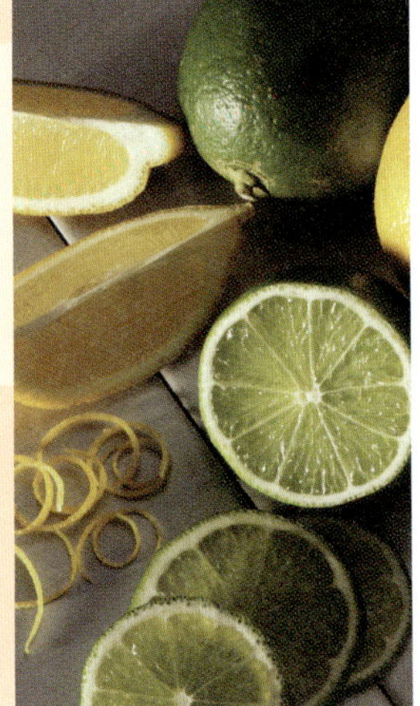

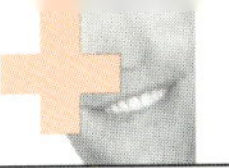

## CIDER VINEGAR

*This is a fermented product derived from apples, which has rejuvenating and curative properties. Helps to keep a healthy level of acids in the body, which tend to plummet when exhausted. Contains calcium, magnesium, sodium, phosphorus, cilium and potassium.*

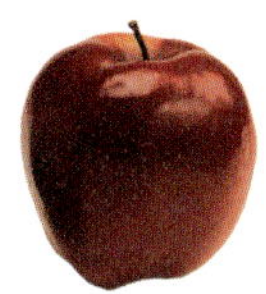

## REFRESHING VINEGAR

Mix 1 glass of water, 2 spoonfuls of cider vinegar and 1 spoon of honey. Mix together and drink small sips. This beverage is recommended for cases of extreme exhaustion and as a daily energizer for athletes.

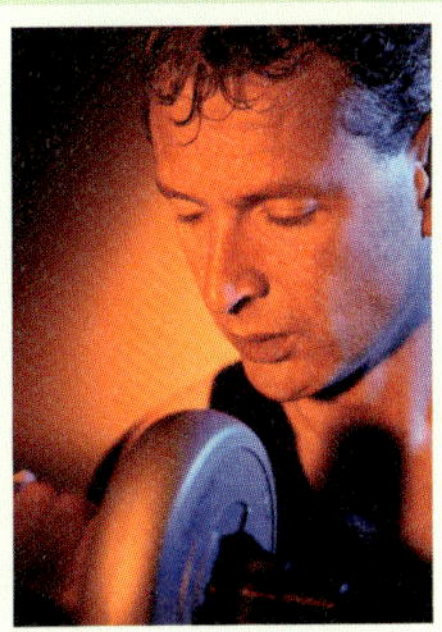

## APRICOTS

Fresh or dried apricots are rich in vitamin C, potassium, fiber, iron and calcium. Dried apricots contain five times more potassium than fresh apricots. It's recommended to eat dried fruits in cases of exhaustion or when exercising. Apricot sauce is recommended when you feel tired, because it contains a high amount of potassium.

## ENERGETIC DOSE FOR WOMEN

**6 dried apricots provide about 13 percent of the recommended daily amount of iron for women. Eating apricots daily helps to energize your body and prevent anaemia.**

## Phosphorus

Found in the body's cells, it is the most abundant mineral in the body after calcium. It is necessary for the chemical reaction in the body to capture, transfer and store energy, for the formation of the bone structure and for the nervous system and brain functions. A lack of phosphorus can cause weakness, mental confusion, loss of appetite, anaemia and general low resistance to

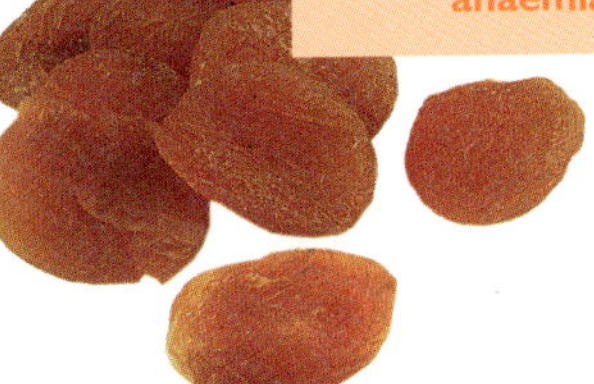

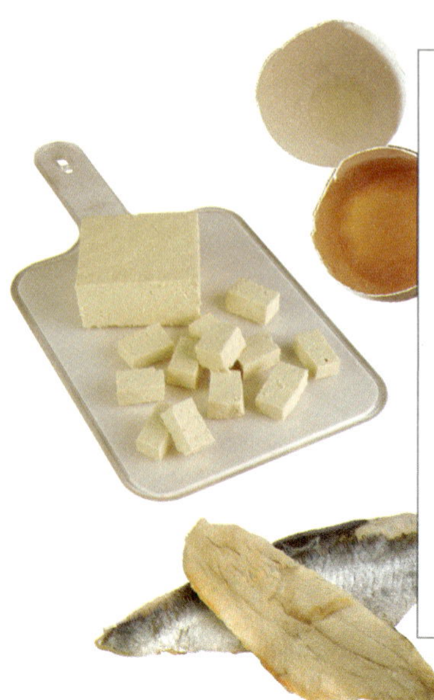

**PHOSPHORUS RICH DIET**

*Any of the following combinations of foods provides the recommended daily dose of phosphorus:*

- *Ample portion of fish, 2 glasses of skim milk;*
- *1 cup of firm tofu, 1 portion of cheese, 1 ham sandwich;*
- *1 portion of lean red meat, 1 egg, 1 portion of cheese;*
- *1 cup of cooked lentils, 1 spoonful of cottage cheese, 1 spoonful of brewers' yeast, 1 egg.*

**ENERGETIC SMOOTHY FOR CHILDREN**

Blend in a blender 4 pears and 2 bananas with powdered milk and sugar. Blend for 2 minutes and serve with crushed ice. This refreshing drink is a yummy treat for kids and all ages.

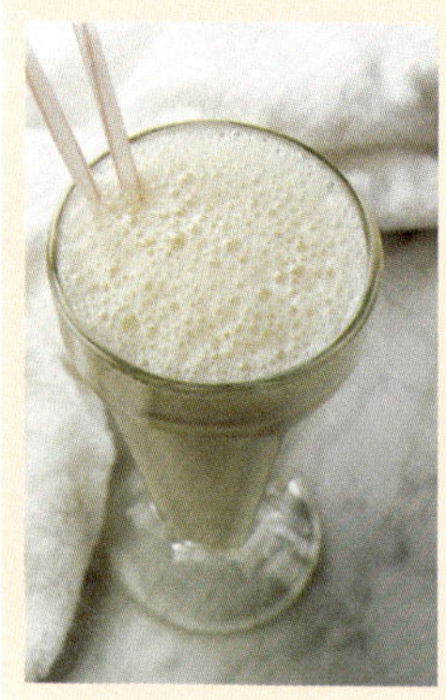

illnesses. Absorption of phosphorus is increased with calcium and vitamin D. Found in **honey**, **white fish**, **brewers' yeast**, **dairy products**, **cereals**, **walnuts**, **figs**, **mushrooms**, **onion** and **cauliflower**.

## Magnesium

Vital for the cellular function that helps the body to produce energy. Supports the muscular and cardiac functions and transmits nervous impulses. It is recommended for cases of exhaustion. Found in **meats**, **walnuts**, **milk**, **maize**, **sesame seeds**, **chestnuts**, **broccoli**, **almonds** and **grapes**.

## Potassium

Provides an essential nutrients for cellular function helping to produce energy in the body, because it helps to stabilize heart rhythm and blood pressure, remove toxins

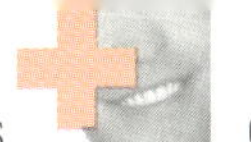

and regulates activity in the intestines and kidneys. It also influences muscle and nervous activity, helping to keep a healthy balance of fluids. Can easily be lost when sweating during physical activities, it is also used as a diuretic. A lack of potassium can cause excessive fatigue, heart palpitations, confusion and depression. Found in **bananas, pears, grapes, apple cider vinegar, salmon** and some **vegetables.**

**PEARS**

**Carbohydrates found in pears are slowly released in the body, which helps to keep up the body's energy level. It's an ideal food for athletes or if you exercise a lot. Contains high levels of potassium, soluble fiber and beta-carotene.**

**It has been proven that the oligo element called boro improves brain activity.**

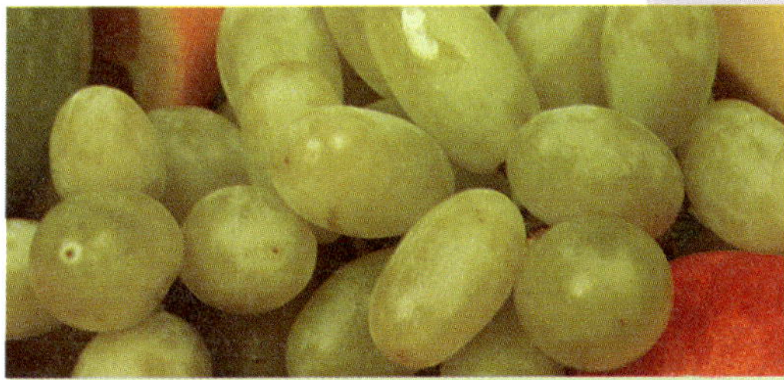

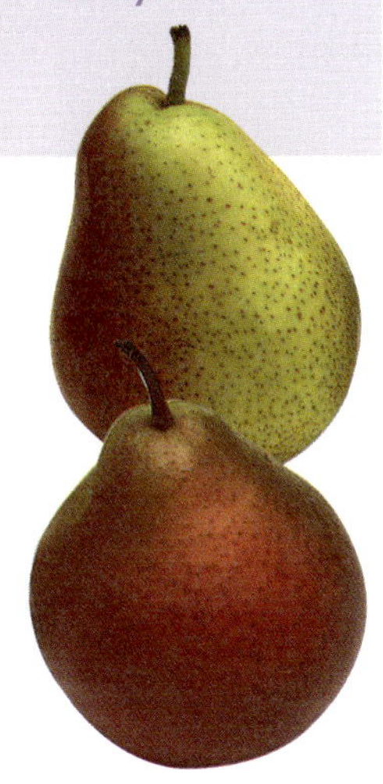

**GRAPES**

Grapes are considered one of the best fruits because their components stimulate neurons, increase vital energy and tone the blood. The main nutrient found in grapes is potassium, but they also contain proteins, sodium, magnesium, iron and phosphorus. With therapeutic effects, it is used as a decoction, juice or ground.

**Safety.** Contain high amounts of sugar. When eaten in excessive amounts can cause feelings of anguish, disillusion and sympthoms of diarrhea. Not recommended for cases of diabetes.

**TONIC FOR VITAL ENERGY**

**Extract grape juice and place over fire until it forms a syrup. Mix with an equal amount of honey, let cool and place in a bottle. Drink 1 tablespoon, mixed with water twice a day.**

# index

## Introduction



## Complementary Therapies



## Natural Herb Remedies



## Healing Foods



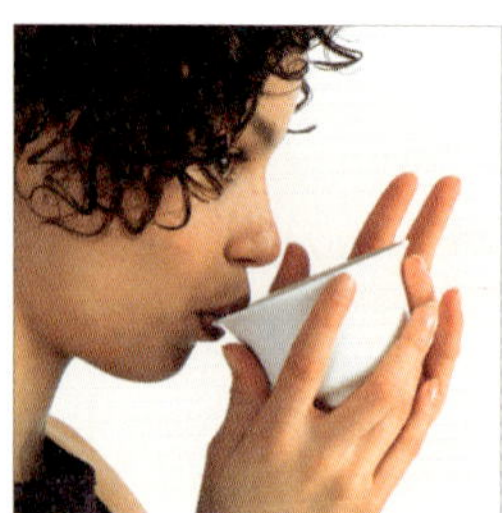